INTERNATIONAL CONGRESS AND SYMPOSIUM SERIES NUMBER 154

Editor-in-Chief: **Hugh L'Etang**

Management of Urinary Tract Infections

Proceedings of an International Consensus Conference sponsored by Norwich Eaton Pharmaceuticals, Inc., held in Montreal, Canada, 11–12 November 1988

Edited by

Lloyd H. Harrison

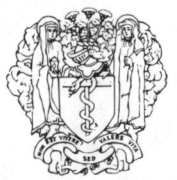

The Bowman Gray School of Medicine designates this continuing medical education activity for 3 credit hours in Category 1 of the Physician's Recognition Award of the American Medical Association

ROYAL SOCIETY OF MEDICINE SERVICES
LONDON · NEW YORK
1990

Royal Society of Medicine Services Limited
1 Wimpole Street   London W1M 8AE
7 East 60th Street   New York NY 10022

©1990 Royal Society of Medicine Services Limited

All rights reserved. No part of this book may be reproduced in any form by photostat, microfilm, or any other means, without written permission from the publishers.

This publication is copyright under the Berne Convention and the International Copyright Convention. All rights reserved. Apart from any fair dealing under the UK Copyright Act 1956, Part 1, Section 7, no part of this publication may be reproduced, stored in a retrieval system or transmitted in any form or by any means without the prior permission of the Honorary Editors, Royal Society of Medicine.

These proceedings are published by Royal Society of Medicine Services Ltd with financial support from the sponsor. The contributors are responsible for the scientific content and for the views expressed, which are not necessarily those of the sponsor, of the editor of the series or of the volume, of the Royal Society of Medicine or of Royal Society of Medicine Services Ltd. Distribution has been in accordance with the wishes of the sponsor but a copy is available to any Fellow of the Society at a privileged price.

Library Cataloging in Publication Data
Management of urinary tract infections
  1. Man. Urinary tract. Diagnosis & therapy
  I. Harrison, L. II. International Congress and
  Symposium Series: ISSN 0142-2367: 154
  616.6

ISBN 1-85315-111-4

Contents developed and produced by
Medical Publishing Enterprises
15–22 Fair Lawn Avenue
Fair Lawn, New Jersey 07410
USA
Phototypeset by Dobbie Typesetting Limited, Plymouth, Devon
Printed in Great Britain at the Alden Press, Oxford

Conference Participants

Editor

L. H. Harrison   Section on Urology, Bowman Gray School of Medicine of Wake Forest University, 300 South Hawthorne Road, Winston-Salem, North Carolina 27103, USA

A. J. Bint   Department of Microbiology, Royal Victoria Infirmary, Newcastle Upon Tyne NE1 4LP, UK

W. Brumfitt   Urinary Infection Clinic, Department of Medical Microbiology, The Royal Free Hospital School of Medicine, Pond Street, Hampstead, London NW3 2OG, UK

E. Calderón-Jaimes   Center for Infectious Disease Research, National Institute of Public Health of Mexico, Lieja No. 7, First Floor, Mexico City, Mexico DS. 06696

M. Elhilali   Department of Urology, Royal Victoria Hospital and McGill University Faculty of Medicine, 3655 Drummond Street, Montreal, Quebec, Canada H3G 1Y6

E. Gomez   National University of Colombia School of Medicine, University City, Section 400, Bogotá, Colombia

G. Harding   Departments of Medicine & Medical Microbiology and Family Practice, University of Manitoba Faculty of Medicine, Winnipeg, Manitoba, Canada R3E OW3

C. C. McOsker   Norwich Eaton Pharmaceuticals, Inc., Woods Corner, Norwich, New York 13815, USA

D. J. Moseley   General Practitioner, Bamford, Near Sheffield S30 2BR, UK

S. G. Mulholland   Department of Urology, Jefferson Medical College of Thomas Jefferson University, 1025 Walnut Street, Philadelphia, Pennsylvania 19107, USA

J. C. Nickel   Department of Urology, Queen's University Faculty of Medicine, Kingston, Ontario, Canada K7L 3N6

C. L. Parsons University of California Medical Center, H-897, 225 Dickinson Street, San Diego, California 92103, USA

P. J. Van Cangh Division of Urology, St Luc University Hospital, 10 Avenue Hippocrate, B-1200 Brussels, Belgium

P. E. V. Van Kerrebroeck Department of Urology, Sint Radboud University Hospital, Geert Grooteplein, Zuid 16, PB9101, NL-6500-HB Nijmegen, The Netherlands

Contents

List of Conference Participants   iii

Differential diagnosis of uncomplicated versus complicated urinary tract infection   1
Lloyd H. Harrison

Selecting therapy for uncomplicated UTI: Viewpoint from the USA   7
C. Lowell Parsons

Selecting therapy for uncomplicated urinary tract infection: A European perspective   15
Paul J. Van Cangh

An open-label randomized comparative trial of nitrofurantoin macrocrystals and TMP-SMX in acute urinary tract infection in Colombia   25
Eugenio Gomez

Inhibition of bacterial protein synthesis by nitrofurantoin macrocrystals: An explanation for the continued efficacy of nitrofurantoin   33
Charles C. McOsker, Jay R. Pollack and Jon A. Andersen

A comparison of amoxicillin, co-trimoxazole, nitrofurantoin macrocrystals, and trimethoprim in the treatment of lower urinary tract infection   45
Ronald Ellis and David J. Moseley

Prospective randomized comparison of the therapeutic efficacy and safety of nitrofurantoin macrocrystals vs norfloxacin in the treatment of acute symptomatic uncomplicated UTIs in women: A preliminary report   53
Godfrey Harding, Lindsay Nicolle, Clare Hawkins, Patricia Mirwaldt and Allan Ronald

Preventive therapy in urinary tract infection: Twenty years' experience   59
William Brumfitt and Jeremy M. T. Hamilton-Miller

Special considerations in the management of acute urinary tract infection   69
Philippe E. V. Van Kerrebroeck

Managing recurrent urinary tract infections   79
S. Grant Mulholland

Special considerations in the management of complicated urinary tract infections   85
J. Curtis Nickel

Women's attitudes and the treatment of urinary tract infections   97
Mostafa Elhilali

Managing uncomplicated urinary tract infections: A worldwide consensus   105
Roundtable Discussion

Continuing Medical Education Test   111

Educational Objectives

After studying these proceedings, the physician will be better able to:

- Evaluate symptoms and diagnose various forms of urinary tract infections (UTIs)
- Select an appropriate treatment for the management of uncomplicated UTIs
- Understand suppressive therapy for UTIs and
- Recognize special considerations in managing acute, recurrent, and complicated UTIs

Publication: January 1990
This program will qualify for 3 hours Category 1 CME credit until February 1992. After that date, tests will be corrected, but CME credit will not be awarded.

Differential diagnosis of uncomplicated versus complicated urinary tract infection

L. H. Harrison

Department of Urology, Bowman Gray School of Medicine of Wake Forest University, Winston-Salem, North Carolina, USA

ABSTRACT

Of the 6 million cases of urinary tract infection (UTI) treated annually by physicians, more than 5 million are acute, simple infections. Simple UTI occurs in anatomically normal urinary tracts, does not promote persistent bacteriuria, and can be easily cured; however, it may recur. The less common, complicated UTI generally involves the upper urinary tract, and can lead to renal damage. Correct diagnosis is necessary for proper management. For women, simple UTI must first be distinguished from other conditions accompanied by dysuria, including vaginitis. Although invasive techniques can differentiate simple from complicated UTI and determine the site of infection, a leukocyte count is the most clinically reliable test. Urinalysis will reveal bacteriuria in both simple and complicated UTI, but urine cultures need not be performed routinely for simple UTI since the majority of infecting organisms are sensitive to antimicrobial treatment.

INTRODUCTION

It is ironic that with all the modern advances in medicine, mankind continues to be bothered by recurrent uncomplicated UTIs. Studies indicate 90% of the 6 million cases of UTIs treated in the physician's office every year are acute and uncomplicated infections (1). *Escherichia coli* accounts for approximately 80% of all UTIs and *Staphylococcus saprophyticus* for 11% (2). With numerous antimicrobial agents available, the choice of a proper antibiotic should be easy, and clearing of the infection simple.

Why then does the uncomplicated UTI continue to be such a problem? The associated morbidity and lost time from work, cost of medications, patient frustration experienced from lower irritative symptoms, and bacterial resistance to antimicrobial therapy and resultant secondary infections are major problems. We know now that uncomplicated urinary infections do not cause renal deterioration, which is a radical change in the perception of recurrent UTIs since the 1960s (3,4). Because of the economic and social burdens caused by uncomplicated UTIs, we have an obligation to take them seriously, thereby treating them promptly and appropriately.

Management of urinary tract infections, edited by Lloyd H. Harrison, 1990; Royal Society of Medicine Services International Congress and Symposium Series No. 154, published by Royal Society of Medicine Services Limited.

Before we can treat an uncomplicated UTI appropriately, we have to ascertain that it is truly an uncomplicated UTI. Therefore, it is important to analyze the nature of these infections thoroughly (5). Proper diagnosis of uncomplicated UTI and selection of appropriate antimicrobial therapy can achieve the cure.

PATHOGENESIS

According to the Food and Drug Administration, complicated UTI is characterized by some condition in the urinary tract known to promote infection, account for persistence of infection, or promote recurrence, which can lead to renal insufficiency (6). With this broad definition given for a complicated UTI, it would appear an uncomplicated UTI could be easily identified as any infection involving the urinary tract that does not promote persistent bacteriuria, i.e., no obstruction, stones, foreign bodies, or fistulae. In other words, an uncomplicated UTI would occur only in anatomically normal urinary tracts and should be easily eradicated (7). Unfortunately, these uncomplicated infections continue to recur frequently in spite of an anatomically normal tract. In fact, recent developments have shown biologic defects are present, and evidence further suggests that of women with recurrent UTIs, increased bacterial adherence to vaginal and transitional epithelium is the norm.

Additionally, certain bacteria seem to have a higher propensity to adhere to the epithelial cells in those women prone to complicated infections than in those considered 'normal' (8). Research has confirmed infection of the urine is preceded by colonization of the vaginal mucosa, followed by adherence of bacteria, and an inflammatory response in the urethra and in the bladder (9), where it is superficial and limited to the epithelium.

Acute infections, either uncomplicated or complicated, can also be subdivided into general anatomic categories: lower tract infection (urethritis, cystitis, and prostatitis) and upper tract infection (acute pyelonephritis) (10). Infections at these sites may occur simultaneously (chronic interstitial nephritis) or independently (cystitis), and may be either asymptomatic or symptomatic. Since bacterial penetration is superficial in a normal urinary tract, cystitis is considered an uncomplicated UTI. In fact, lower urinary tract infections (LUTIs) are generally considered to be uncomplicated. Upper tract infections are complicated because they involve not only infection of the pelvic epithelium but also manifest deep renal parenchymal penetration. Some physicians consider acute pyelonephritis and prostatitis to be uncomplicated in those individuals who have no source of persistent bacteriuria. However, deep tissue penetration moves these infections into the complicated group. Remember that uncomplicated infections do not lead to renal damage even when they recur frequently.

CLINICAL PRESENTATION

History

Close attention to the patient's presenting symptoms allows the physician to differentiate between uncomplicated and complicated UTI. Young, healthy women who come in complaining of dysuria, frequency, urgency, and suprapubic tenderness alert physicians that the condition is most likely an uncomplicated UTI. In addition, the patient may not have a history of UTIs or this may be her first episode in a while (she has had less than three per year, usually with a month or so in between). For appropriate management, LUTI in the woman must be differentiated from other inflammatory or infectious conditions in which dysuria may be the most prominent symptom, such as vaginitis, urethral infections caused by sexually transmitted pathogens, and miscellaneous noninflammatory causes of urethral discomfort (e.g., malignancy). Close attention to characteristic features of the patient's history, the physical examination, and voided urine or other specimens allows patients with dysuria to be assigned to one of these diagnostic categories (11).

The older man who has some causes of persistent bacteriuria, such as a foreign body, obstruction, stone, or fistula, is usually in a more distressed condition. He may have flank pain, malaise, fever, dehydration, nausea, and vomiting and will have a clear indication of a complicated UTI (6).

Physical examination

Typically, the physical examination results of a patient with an uncomplicated UTI are negative, and suprapubic discomfort is usually observed in only 10% of individuals (12). In a patient with a complicated UTI, symptoms may be present with flank tenderness, malaise, and signs of impending sepsis. Each episode of infection must be managed individually by considering the presentation, past history of infection, recent antimicrobial therapy, and presumed or documented infecting organism.

LABORATORY TESTS

The clinical differentiation of complicated and uncomplicated UTIs, is not very reliable. The natural history and therapeutic outcome of a UTI depends on the site of infection within the genitourinary tract. Some clinicians consider localization studies to be very important for proper treatment and prognostic indicators of long-term outlook. Localization of infection to the bladder or kidney may be useful in determining the optimal management of those patients who are experiencing recurrent infection. The most accurate localizing study is bilateral ureteral catheterization (13) for urinalysis and culture. This method requires cystoscopic insertion of ureteral catheters and is too invasive and expensive for routine clinical use.

Another invasive method is the bladder wash-out technique (14), which involves irrigation of the bladder with an antibiotic solution followed by urine collection through a Foley catheter. Positive urine cultures represent upper tract infection because the ureters were the source of the urine. The bladder wash-out technique is too complex for a routine clinical test.

Antibody-coated-bacteria tests (15) used for location unfortunately give a 16% to 18% false-negative result and are primarily useful for research (1). These tests use antibody-coated bacteria recovered from the urine of patients with complicated UTIs. They can be visualized when exposed to fluorescein-labeled antihuman globulin. Bacteria isolated from uncomplicated UTIs show no evidence of antibody coating on their bacterial surfaces. False-positive results in uncomplicated UTIs are less common, and they can be caused by prostatitis, hemorrhagic cystitis, and contamination of the midstream urine with vaginal or bowel organisms.

Other tests, such as assay for C-reactive protein (16), are not diagnostic since elevated results also occur in other infections. A temporary defect in renal concentration ability (17) may be seen in complicated UTIs but is of little use in the day-to-day practice of medicine. Some investigators (18,19) have advocated single-dose antimicrobial therapy as the best localization study and therapy for uncomplicated UTIs in females. Single-dose therapy fails to cure complicated UTI in the majority of cases and some studies indicate patients with uncomplicated UTIs treated with single-dose therapy have more relapses than those undergoing longer treatment. We hope that in the near future, a simple, noninvasive, cost-effective, and accurate test will be devised for the differentiation or localization of uncomplicated (usually lower tract) UTIs versus complicated (usually upper tract) UTIs.

The most consistent laboratory test that, in my opinion, can be used by the attending physician to confirm or predict a complicated UTI, is a blood leukocyte test. Elevation with a shift to the immature cells substantiates possible renal involvement. The white cell count is seen as normal with an uncomplicated UTI. The fastest test for the detection of bacteria and leukocytes is a direct microscopic examination of fresh or gram-stained urine (urinalysis); it can be performed by the attending physician while the patient waits. A urinalysis, in both uncomplicated and complicated UTIs, would demonstrate white blood cells, red blood cells, and bacteriuria if they were present. The presence of bacteriuria on a gram-stained, uncentrifuged, freshly voided urine specimen usually indicates a colony count of greater than 10^5/ml (5,20). In unspun, freshly voided urine with colony counts between 10^2 and 10^4/ml, bacteriuria may not be seen on microscopic examination. Urine cultures are not performed routinely in simple UTI since the majority of organisms usually present in this condition (*E. coli* and other Enterobacteriaceae) are generally sensitive to the antimicrobial agents currently available for treatment.

In complicated UTIs, urine cultures and tests of microbiologic sensitivities are routinely performed. The cultured organisms are quite often resistant to most oral antibiotics. In the majority of colony counts from patients with simple or complicated UTIs, the count is usually greater than 10^5/ml. Approximately one third of uncomplicated UTIs will have colony counts of less than 10^5/ml (usually 10^2 to 10^4). These patients should be treated with appropriate antimicrobial therapy (21).

SUMMARY

I have defined an uncomplicated urinary tract infection as a superficial infection involving the urinary tract, in which there are no obstructions, stones, foreign bodies, or fistulae (normal anatomic urinary tract) and which, thus, does not promote persistent bacteriuria. Once a diagnosis is made, the next clinical question pertains to treatment and prophylactic therapy. Will we continue utilizing accepted therapeutic regimens, i.e., nitrofurantoin (Macrodantin®), which has proved to be cost-effective, to have minimal side effects, and to have a high clinical cure rate? Will new, more powerful agents take its place, or is there an appropriate place in our practice for both types of agents?

Since the majority of UTIs are uncomplicated, it is appropriate that most of the papers in this conference focus on developing a worldwide consensus approach to effective treatment of simple UTIs. However, we should bear in mind that the key to successful treatment is an accurate differential diagnosis of uncomplicated versus complicated UTI.

REFERENCES

(1) Stamm WE, Turck M. Urinary tract infection, pyelonephritis, and related conditions. In: Braunwald E, ed. *Harrison's principles of internal medicine*, 11th ed. New York: McGraw-Hill Book Company, 1987; **225**: 1189–1195.
(2) Latham RH, Running K, Stamm WE. Urinary tract infections in young adult women caused by *Staphylococcus saprophyticus*. *JAMA* 1983; **250**: 3063–3066.
(3) Stamey TA. Recurrent urinary tract infections in female patients: an overview of management and treatment. *Rev Infect Dis* 1987; **9** (suppl 2): S195–210.
(4) Freedman LR. Natural history of urinary infection in adults. *Kidney Int* 1975; **4**: S96–100.
(5) Johnson JR, Stamm WE. Diagnosis and treatment of acute urinary tract infections. *Infect Dis Clin North Am* 1987; **1**: 773–791.
(6) Preheim LC. Complicated urinary tract infections. *Am J Med* 1985; **79**: 62–66.
(7) Kunin CM. An overview of urinary tract infections. In: Kunin CM, ed. *Detection, prevention and management of urinary tract infections*. Philadelphia: Lea & Febiger, 1987; **1**: 1–55.
(8) Parsons CL. Lower urinary tract infections in women. *Urol Clin North Am* 1987; **14**: 247–250.
(9) Schaeffer AJ. Pathogenesis of recurrent urinary tract infection: use of understanding as therapy. *Urology* 1988; **32**: 13–16.
(10) Shea DJ. Pyelonephritis and female urinary tract infection. *Emerg Med Clin North Am* 1988; **6**: 403–417.
(11) Berg AO, Soman MP. Lower genitourinary infections in women. *J Fam Pract* 1986; **23**: 61–67.
(12) Wong ES, Fennell CL, Stamm WE. Urinary tract infection among women attending a clinic for sexually transmitted diseases. *Sex Transm Dis* 1984; **11**: 18–23.
(13) Stamey TA. Diagnosis, localization and classification of urinary infection. In: *Pathogenesis and treatment of urinary tract infections*. Baltimore: Williams & Wilkins Co, 1980; **I**: 1–51.
(14) Fairley KF, Bond AG, Brown RB, Habersberger P. Simple test to determine the site of urinary-tract infection. *Lancet* 1967; **ii**: 427–428.
(15) Thomas V, Shelokov A, Forland M. Antibody-coated bacteria in the urine and the site of urinary tract infection. *N Engl J Med* 1975; **290**: 588–590.
(16) Fierer J. Acute pyelonephritis. *Urol Clin North Am* 1987; **14**: 251–256.
(17) Ronald AR, Cutler RE, Turck M. Effect of bacteriuria on renal concentrating mechanisms. *Ann Intern Med* 1969; **70**: 723–733.
(18) Turck M. New concepts in genitourinary tract infections. *JAMA* 1981; **246**: 2019–2023.
(19) Schultz HJ, McCaffrey LA, Keys TF, Nobrega FT. Acute cystitis: a prospective study of laboratory tests and duration of therapy. *Mayo Clin Proc* 1984; **59**: 391–397.
(20) Jenkins RD, Fenn JP, Matsen JM. Review of urine microscopy for bacteriuria. *JAMA* 1986; **255**: 3397–3403.
(21) Tolkoff-Rubin NE, Rubin RH. New approaches to the treatment of urinary tract infection. *Am J Med* 1987; **82**: 270–277.

Selecting therapy for uncomplicated UTI: Viewpoint from the USA

C. L. Parsons

University of California Medical Center, San Diego, California, USA

ABSTRACT

Faced with a multitude of therapeutic choices for the treatment of uncomplicated acute and recurrent urinary tract infection (UTI), the clinician must respond by deriving rational criteria to guide the selection. Four criteria must be considered when selecting a first-line therapy. First, an antibiotic must attain adequate concentrations in the urine. Second, the agent of choice should have a minimal effect on normal flora in the intestine and third, on normal flora in the vagina, thereby preventing unnecessary resistance or yeast vaginitis, and reinfection. Resistance to drugs with broad tissue distribution is a concern, as agents used in UTIs may also be useful in other, non-urinary-tract infections, which are more difficult to treat. Fourth, agents with a low total cost are preferred for routine use. Two currently available antibiotics for use in acute UTI most closely meet these criteria: nitrofurantoin macrocrystals (Macrodantin®) and penicillin VK. For routine use, the clinician should consider one of these agents first, avoiding possible hypersensitivity reactions where they may be a concern.

INTRODUCTION

Many therapeutic choices are available for the treatment of uncomplicated urinary tract infection (UTI), including agents from a number of different antibiotic classes. All of these drugs are effective in most cases of acute, uncomplicated UTI. However, many of these agents are associated with significant effects on the normal flora of the vagina and intestine, frequently leading to unnecessary complications such as yeast vaginitis, recurrent infections, and the generation of resistant strains of bacteria (1–3). Significant differences are also seen in cost, an issue of steadily increasing importance. In particular patients, of course, drug sensitivies may limit the choice of therapy. Faced with a multitude of choices, the clinician must determine which antibiotics meet the ideal criteria and prescribe a low-cost antibiotic that does not cause unacceptable side effects.

AMERICAN MEDICAL PRACTICE AND THE TREATMENT OF UTI

Several important economic and sociologic changes in America have profoundly affected the practice of medicine. The most evident and far-reaching change is the increased emphasis on cost containment. An estimated 6% to 8% of young women contract a UTI annually, resulting in 5.2 million office visits. At approximately $140 per treatment, this approaches a yearly cost of $1 billion (4,5).

Pressure to reduce this cost comes not only from the patient but also from a variety of private and government third-party payers who are responsible for financing the medical bills of most Americans. Health maintenance organizations are particularly active in applying cost-control measures. One response to these pressures has been to reconsider the need for routine urine cultures (6).

A second response has been the use of shorter durations of therapy, which are effective, cost less, and may reduce the rate of side effects. Of course, one has to be cautious not to shorten the course of therapy too much or the infection may not clear completely. For the patient, the total cost of each episode of infection includes resolution of morbidity as well as the cost of an office visit and therapy for a second try.

For some patients, a three-day full course of therapy, followed by single night-time doses for four nights may be an effective compromise (5). However, in many cases the physician may be more comfortable with the traditional seven-to-10 day course of therapy. When considering cost, it is important to recognize the true cost of therapy, which may go well beyond the cost of the initial office visit and purchase price of the medication. In UTI, the costs of return visits and/or additional medications necessitated by failure, recurrence of the infections, or drug side effects, such as yeast vaginitis, will ultimately be much greater than the cost of the initial prescription.

Another major change in American medicine is the increasing tendency of patients to view themselves as health-care consumers, rather than the doctor's patient. They are more knowledgeable about potential therapies and may wish to be involved in decisions about their care. At the same time, the busy life-styles and careers of most American women, combined with the progress of medical science, have created an expectation of 'perfect' treatment that will rapidly cure infection, will not cause side effects, and most especially will not require additional medications or a return visit. Given the joint pressures of cost containment and patient expectations, the importance of prescribing an antibiotic with minimal potential for recurrent infections or other troublesome side effects becomes even more obvious.

CRITERIA FOR SELECTING AN ANTIBIOTIC

Four criteria can be used for selecting an antibiotic to treat UTIs. As shown in Table 1, these are high urinary levels, minimal effects on intestinal microflora, minimal effects on vaginal microflora, and low total cost.

High urinary levels

The most obvious, and most easily met, requirement is the attainment of high antibiotic levels in the urine and bladder. The primary pathogen of concern, of course, is *Escherichia coli*, with enterococcus the next most frequent isolate (4,7,8). For the most part, the oral antibiotics commonly used in uncomplicated UTI are

Table 1 *Criteria for selecting antibiotics for routine treatment of uncomplicated UTI*

1. High urinary levels for bactericidal efficacy
2. Minimal effects on intestinal microflora to help avoid resistance
   (High gastrointestinal absorption)
3. Minimal effects on vaginal microflora to avoid unnecessary side effects
   (Low serum levels)
4. Low cost

active against both of these pathogens at the levels obtained in the urine. However, significant resistance to sulfonamides and penicillins such as amoxicillin—in the range of 25% to 35%—has been reported with *E. coli* strains, even in community-acquired UTI (4,5). An additional issue concerns activity against enterococci. Although enterococci are infrequent in initial infections, they occur much more frequently in recurrent UTI, presumably because they are selected by antibiotics (particularly cephalosporins) lacking antienterococcal activity (9).

Minimal effect on intestinal flora

Of the remaining factors to consider, the most important is the impact on the normal intestinal flora. In practice, this suggests avoiding antibiotics with poor gastrointestinal absorption, although high serum levels also cause such effects (10). While the proximate source of bacteria in acute UTI may be the vagina or perineum, the fecal flora are almost always the ultimate source of *E. coli* strains in UTI (11). This becomes important for the 20% of outpatients who will develop recurrent infections. Drugs that strongly alter the normal flora of the gut select for resistant microbes. These resistant pathogens may then cause infections recalcitrant to the original drug or to other antibiotics of the same class. Disturbances of gut flora also lead to diarrhea, which potentially can decrease compliance or necessitate drug discontinuation. Ampicillin, tetracycline, and trimethoprim-sulfamethoxazole (TMP-SMX) are examples of drugs with high stool effects. The use of broadly distributed antibiotics with marked effects on intestinal flora for chronic or suppressive therapy particularly should be avoided, since that would lengthen the time available for resistant strains to arise.

Minimal effect on vaginal flora

The choice of an antibiotic that produces low serum levels is also important to lessen the effect on vaginal microflora. Changes in the normal vaginal environment frequently cause yeast overgrowth. With some antibiotics, such as ampicillin, this is seen in as many as 25% of patients (12). These infections can be even more difficult and costly to treat than the initial UTI. They upset the patient and require additional visits to the physician's office. Furthermore, the effects of antimycotics to treat vaginal candidiasis may in turn lead to bacterial overgrowth and bacterial vaginitis, if the antibiotic has been discontinued. The disruption of normal bacterial flora (mostly lactobacilli) also promotes colonization of the vagina by coliform bacteria. Studies have demonstrated that many recurrent infections actually represent infections by fecal flora that have colonized the vagina, rather than failure to clear the initial infection (13–17). Therefore, a decrease in effect on vaginal microflora might be expected to reduce the rate of recurrence.

Cost

The final major criterion is cost. In today's cost-conscious environment, the physician should select the least expensive antibiotic available that meets the therapeutic goals. Newer antibiotics are more expensive than older ones, so it is up to the individual prescriber to determine whether they offer compensating clinical advantages relevant to a particular patient. In addition, limiting the use of newer, more costly antibiotics not only reduces cost but also allows the clinician additional time in which to evaluate the drugs' safety profiles in actual clinical use before using them more widely.

Ironically, because many of our pharmacists charge a dispensing fee, it can be cost-effective to prescribe a seven-to-10 day course of therapy. It can be very expensive if you prescribe only a few pills and the patient has to return to the pharmacy for another prescription.

EVALUATION OF CURRENTLY AVAILABLE ANTIBIOTICS

Using these criteria, one may arbitrarily assign points to punish a drug should it have a high cost, vaginal vault effects, or clonic flora effects. When this is done and the points are totalled, the antibiotics will align themselves in a list that can be divided into five categories. It is suggested that the clinician select the highest-rated, well-tolerated antibiotic, being particularly careful when hypersensitivity is a concern. These classes, together with doses frequently used in treating uncomplicated UTI, are shown in Table 2.

Class 1

There are two antibiotics in class 1: nitrofurantoin macrocrystals (Macrodantin®) and penicillin VK. Nitrofurantoin macrocrystals achieve high bactericidal urine concentrations against the most common urinary tract pathogens: *E. coli*, enterococci, and *Staphylococcus saprophyticus*. Because all forms of nitrofurantoin

Table 2 *Commonly prescribed antibiotics for uncomplicated UTIs*

	Usual dose
Class 1	
Nitrofurantoin macrocrystals	50 mg q.i.d.
Penicillin VK	250 mg q.i.d.
Class 2	
Sulfonamides	500 mg q.i.d.
Carbenicillin	500 mg t.i.d.
Class 3	
Amoxicillin	250 mg t.i.d.
Class 4	
Trimethoprim-sulfamethoxazole	360 mg/120 mg b.i.d.
Cephalexin	250 mg t.i.d.
Cefadroxil	500 mg b.i.d.
Class 5	
Ampicillin	250 mg t.i.d.
Tetracycline	250 mg q.i.d.
Norfloxacin	400 mg b.i.d.
Ciprofloxacin	250 mg b.i.d.

are well absorbed from the intestine, reduced efficacy due to resistance among strains of previously confirmed susceptible pathogens is essentially unknown, even though 30 years have passed since the drug's introduction (18). Recent data suggest that the unique bactericidal mode of action of nitrofurantoin also contributes to this lack of resistance (19). Nitrofurantoin macrocrystals have a serum half-life of approximately 20 min in normal patients and are metabolized in many tissues in the body. Its effect on vaginal flora is negligible and the rate of yeast vaginitis with this drug is exceptionally low.

The combination of these properties makes nitrofurantoin macrocrystals an ideal first-line choice for treating uncomplicated UTI. Microcrystalline nitrofurantoin is less well tolerated. Compared with the macrocrystalline product, microcrystalline nitrofurantoin may cause significant nausea and vomiting, leading to decreased patient compliance and an increased risk of persistence or recurrence of infections that were treated for inadequate time periods. Consequently, the macrocrystalline form is preferable for clinical use, as it has a better tolerance profile. In fact, the macrocrystals, when taken with meals, provides increased absorption while further increasing gastrointestinal tolerance. The compliance advantage of the macrocrystalline form is especially important in chronic, suppressive therapy, since patients not suffering from the symptoms of acute infection are less likely to comply with a medicine causing uncomfortable side effects.

Penicillin VK is another class 1 antibiotic and another good choice for uncomplicated UTI. It is a class 1 drug because of its low cost, low effects on vaginal/colonic flora, and its bactericidal urinary concentration against *E. coli* and enterococci; it is usually not active against staphylococci. Unfortunately, this drug must generally be used empirically, since clinical laboratories often do not test for susceptibility at the concentrations achieved in the urine.

Class 2

The first group of class 2 antibiotics are the sulfonamides, including sulfisoxazole and sulfamethoxazole. Both have been used for many years, and they are still viable options for lower UTI. However, they have also been long recognized as contributing to the development of resistant pathogens in the bowel (1,3). For this reason, they are not indicated for long-term or suppressive therapy. Carbenicillin meets the designated therapeutic criteria and adds activity against *Proteus mirabilis* and *Pseudomonas aeruginosa*. However, these pathogens are very infrequent in uncomplicated UTI. Furthermore, carbenicillin is significantly more costly than the class 1 drugs and the sulfonamides.

Class 3

Amoxicillin is well absorbed and attains high urine concentrations. The primary disadvantage of amoxicillin for management of urinary tract infections is its high serum levels. As a result, up to 25% of patients on amoxicillin develop yeast vaginitis (20).

Class 4

The agents in this class tend to have several significant drawbacks, such as high vaginal vault effects, problems with resistance in the intestinal flora, and a higher cost than other antibiotics—for example, penicillin VK. Among them,

TMP-SMX (known in many countries as co-trimoxazole) and oral cephalosporins are well absorbed and clinically effective against common pathogens. Effects on vaginal flora are moderate (less than those of amoxicillin), but recent data suggest increasing levels of resistance in the intestinal flora (3). Furthermore, although the cost has come down, these agents are among the more expensive oral antibiotics available, making them a reserve choice in most situations. In fact, in the United States, even the manufacturers of TMP-SMX recommend on their package inserts that it be reserved as second-line therapy.

TMP-SMX and oral cephalosporins offer an expanded spectrum of activity against gram-negative bacteria (including *Klebsiella* sp and *P. mirabilis*). On the other hand, gram-negative bacteria other than *E. coli* are infrequent in community practice and rare in uncomplicated UTI in otherwise healthy young women. These antibiotics are more appropriately used after other antibiotics fail, when cultures indicate the presence of unusual organisms, or in elderly patients with risk factors suggesting the presence of abnormal gram-negative pathogens.

Class 5

Two members of class 5, ampicillin and tetracycline have little, if anything, to recommend them in contemporary practice for the treatment of UTI. Both are very poorly absorbed, with levels in the feces actually up to three times those in the urine (21). This high antibiotic level has significant deleterious effects on the normal intestinal microflora. These effects are associated with significant resistance problems to both drugs. In addition, with these drugs, as with amoxicillin, rates of yeast vaginitis approach 25%.

The other class 5 antibiotics are the new fluoroquinolones, norfloxacin, and ciprofloxacin. Each offers high potency and a very broad spectrum, comparable to many injectable antibiotics. However, these broad spectra are of little relevance to the treatment of uncomplicated UTI in typical patients. At the same time, there are very significant safety concerns attendant with the use of fluoroquinolones in women of childbearing age; these agents are contraindicated in children and in pregnant women because of their damaging effects on cartilage development. For this reason, their use should be reserved, which may also delay the development of resistance to these agents (preserving their activity against strains resistant to other antibiotics). Additionally, reserving their use allows practitioners time to observe their safety profiles in routine clinical use. Last, these drugs, while cost-effective alternatives to parenteral antibiotics, are far more expensive when compared with other time-proven oral antibiotics more appropriately used to treat simple cystitis and other common community-acquired UTIs.

CONCLUSION

The imperatives of contemporary American medical practice require that the clinician prescribes therapy that will be not only effective in relieving the condition but also convenient for the patient. The desire to avoid side effects has always been part of standard medical practice, and this leads to an even greater recognition of the importance of the four criteria: achieving high urine concentrations, preventing disruption of the normal vaginal and intestinal floras, and providing all at low cost. Emphasis on cost containment has greatly increased.

Thus, antibiotics selected for uncomplicated UTI must not only meet these four criteria but also should be well absorbed, provide low serum concentrations, be well tolerated, and be cost-effective. The physician should consider first the highest rated drug to which the patient is not sensitive. By using these criteria, the two antibiotics best suited for routine treatment of simple cystitis and other forms of uncomplicated UTIs are nitrofurantoin macrocrystals and penicillin VK.

REFERENCES

(1) Parsons CL. Lower urinary tract infections in women. *Urol Clin North Am* 1987; **14**: 247–250.
(2) Winberg J. Urinary tract infections in infants and children. In: Harrison J, Gittes R, Perlmutter A, eds. *Campbell's urology*, 4th ed. Philadelphia: WB Saunders Co., 1978; **1**: 481.
(3) Schaeffer AJ. Recurrent urinary tract infection in the female patient. *Urology* 1988; **32** (suppl 3): 12–15.
(4) Iravani A. Bacterial infections of the urinary tract—female. In: Rakel RE, ed. *Conn's current therapy*. Philadelphia: WB Saunders Co., 1987: 538–541.
(5) Johnson JR, Stamm WE. Diagnosis and treatment of acute urinary tract infections. *Infect Dis Clin North Am* 1987; **1**: 773–791.
(6) Stamm WE. When should we use urine cultures? *Infect Control* 1986; **7**: 431–433.
(7) Corriere JN, Hanno PM, Hooton T. Cystitis: evolving standard of care. *Patient Care* 1988; **29**: 33–47.
(8) Wilhelm MP, Edson RS. Antimicrobial agents in urinary tract infections. *Mayo Clin Proc* 1987; **63**: 1025–1031.
(9) Norrby SR. Principles for targeted antibiotic use in urinary tract and enteric infections: a review with special emphasis on norfloxacin. *Scand J Infect Dis* 1986; **48** (suppl): 7–19.
(10) Parsons CL. Antibiotic selection for lower urinary tract infections. *Fam Pract Recert* 1987; **9** (suppl): 9.
(11) Schaeffer AJ. Recurrent urinary tract infection in women. Pathogenesis and management. *Postgrad Med* 1987; **8**: 51–58.
(12) Buchsbaum HJ, Schmidt JD. *Gynecologic and obstetric urology*, 2nd ed. Philadelphia: WB Saunders Co., 1982; **24**: 347–72.
(13) Stamey TA, Kaufman MF. Studies of introital colonization in women with recurrent urinary infections. II. A comparison of growth in normal vaginal fluid of common versus uncommon serogroups of *Escherichia coli*. *J Urol* 1975; **114**: 264–267.
(14) Stamey TA, Sexton CC. The role of vaginal colonization with Enterobacteriaceae in recurrent urinary infections. *J Urol* 1975; **113**: 214–217.
(15) Stamey TA, Timothy MM. Studies of introital colonization in women with recurrent urinary tract infections. I. The role of vaginal pH. *J Urol* 1976; **114**: 261–263.
(16) Stamey TA, Timothy M, Miller M, *et al*. Recurrent urinary tract infections in adult women: the role of introital enterobacteria. *California Medicine* 1971; **115**: 1.
(17) Schaeffer AJ, Jones JM, Dunn JK. Association of *in vitro Escherichia coli* adherence to vaginal and buccal epithelial cells with susceptibility of women to recurrent urinary-tract infections. *N Engl J Med* 1981; **304**: 1062–1066.
(18) McCall DR. Nitrofurans. In: Hahn FE, ed. *Mechanism of action of antimicrobial agents*. New York: Springer-Verlag, 1979: 176.
(19) McOsker CC, Pollack JR, Andersen JA. Inhibition of bacterial protein synthesis by nitrofurantoin macrocrystals: An explanation for the continued efficacy of nitrofurantoin. *Royal Society of Medicine Services International Congress and Symposium Series*. This volume, 33–44.
(20) Parsons CL. Protocol for treatment of typical urinary tract infection: criteria for antimicrobial selection. *Urology* 1988; **32** (suppl): 22–27.
(21) Knudsen ET, Rolinson G, Stevens S. Absorption and excretion of 'Penbriten'. *Br Med J* 1962; **2**: 198.

Selecting therapy for uncomplicated urinary tract infection: A European perspective

P. J. Van Cangh

Division of Urology, St Luc University Hospital, Brussels, Belgium

ABSTRACT

Antibiotic selection for urinary tract infection (UTI) encompasses several factors, including microorganism specificity, side effects, and total cost. In Belgium, norfloxacin, minocycline, and amoxicillin-clavulanic acid are the most expensive antibiotics on a per dose basis; nitrofurantoin macrocrystals (Macrodantin®) is one of the least expensive. Medication is priced on a sliding scale based on income, hence patients do not bear full costs of their medication. Initial findings of a urinary pathogen study conducted by St Luc University Hospital in Brussels reveal a high incidence of *Escherichia coli* resistance to amoxicillin, ampicillin, and trimethoprim/sulfamethoxazole. Resistance to nitrofurantoin macrocrystals is extremely low. This low resistance along with the drug's urinary tract specificity, enables nitrofurantoin to remain the most widely prescribed antimicrobial agent for urinary tract infections in this country.

HEALTH CARE IN WESTERN EUROPE

Health care delivery in Western Europe, especially in the European Economic Community (EEC), or common market, countries, includes a highly developed Social Security system. All individuals are covered by Social Security, as well as by some kind of compulsory health insurance (1).

In Belgium, outpatient medications are classified into three categories (A, B, C) according to their importance; the cost to the patient is directly related to the assigned category (1). The bulk of the cost of essential medications, including antibiotics and most antimicrobials, is borne by the system. Therefore, the real cost of a specific medication has only moderate importance for a specific patient, as he has to disburse only a moderate amount directly. Cost may become a problem, however, in cases of chronic or recurrent infections.

Table 1 lists the 'public price' of the common medications used in Belgium (cost of prescription, and cost for one dose). For these medications, the patient pays out of pocket from 15%—for special social categories: widow, orphan, handicapped, and retired people—to 25% (general population) of the public price (2).

Table 1 *'Public price' of common antibiotics in Belgium*

	Prescription	Cost (BEF)[a]	Cost/dose (BEF)[a]
Nitrofurantoin macrocrystals	50×50 mg	230	5
Nifurtoinol	50×200	350	7
Co-trimaxozole sulfamethoxazole 800 plus trimethoprim (160)	30	388	13
Pipemidic acid	40×200	612	15
Nalidixic acid	28×1000 mg	612	16
Cinoxacin	20×500	612	30
Amoxicillin	16×500 mg	450–600	33
Cephalexin	16×500 mg	532	33
Oxolinic acid	14×750	612	44
Amoxicillin (500) plus clavulanic acid (125)	16	780	49
Minocycline	15×100 mg	777	52
Norfloxacin	6×400	364	61

[a] *1 US dollar = 40 Belgian francs (BEF).*
(Data from reference 16.)

Society, however, is responsible for the financial equilibrium of the system, in that deficits in Social Security must be covered by new taxes. At the present time, a high cost consciousness exists and physicians will usually select the less expensive drug, provided it is equally effective.

The socioeconomic level in the EEC countries is high, and most patients have access to satisfactory health care. Income level has virtually no influence on this because people with lower income pay less for their medical treatments.

Although no scientific study exists, it appears likely that the level of education affects compliance of the patient. In our opinion, persons with a higher education level seek medical help sooner and are more likely to follow their prescriptions. This is particularly important in once-daily treatment, where a missed dose can significantly compromise therapy.

Typical patients with uncomplicated urinary tract infection (UTI) are probably similar all over the world and are most widely represented by women with acute cystitis. The problem is important in magnitude; it is commonly estimated that 20% of all women will have at least one episode of acute lower UTI in their lifetimes (3). A study in Britain reports that 8% of all urban general practitioner visits are motivated by such problems (3).

Usually the patient will seek prompt nonspecialized medical advice, especially for the first acute symptomatic episode. Ten percent of patients with an isolated episode of acute cystitis are referred to the urologist, and 20% of those with recurrent infections. In cases of frequently recurring infections, patients usually see a urologist and, after a negative workup, will probably start on a self-medication program or a low-dose, long-term regimen (2).

SPECTRUM OF UTI PATHOGENS AND PRINCIPLES OF ANTIMICROBIAL THERAPY

In the general population, 80% of uncomplicated UTIs are caused by *E. coli*, and the rest by various organisms including enterococci and coagulase-negative *Staphylococcus* (4,5). Table 2 shows the incidence of urinary pathogens in the

Table 2 *Percent distribution of urinary pathogens*

	Community First UTI	Community Recurrent UTI	University Hospital, Brussels
Escherichia coli	84	75	50
Proteus mirabilis	7	—	9
Proteus/Providencia	—	7	6
Enterococcus	5	5	10
Klebsiella	2	8	8
Staphylococcus, coagulase-negative	1	—	1
Serratia	—	—	1
Enterobacter	—	—	4
Pseudomonas aeruginosa	—	—	9
Others	1	5	2

general population (first episode and recurrent UTI), and in St Luc University Hospital (6,7). Ninety percent of UTIs in the general population are caused by enterobacteriaceae and 10% by gram-positive organisms (mainly enterococci and coagulase-negative *Staphylococcus*). In our university hospital, the spectrum of uropathogens is, not unexpectedly, quite different. Only 50% are *E. coli*, and the rest include various nosocomial pathogens.

Table 3 shows the susceptibility of common uropathogens in two large Belgian multicenter studies and in our university hospital (6,7,8). *E. coli* resistance to ampicillin in the 1985 multicenter studies was 41%, and it was 42% in the hospital study, which was conducted during the period from 1986 to 1988. In the 1985 multicenter study, 4% of *E. coli* infections were resistant to the combination of amoxicillin and clavulanic acid, while in the 1988 multicenter study, 15.7% were resistant (7). Furthermore, in the 1988 study, 17.7% of the infecting strains showed only intermediate sensitivity to this treatment. Our own findings at St Luc University Hospital have confirmed that 8% of the strains are resistant to this combination, and 5% have intermediate sensitivity. *E. coli* resistance to trimethoprim-sulfamethoxazole (TMP-SMX) was 27% in the 1985 multicenter studies and 21% in the hospital study. Resistance of *E. coli* to nitrofurans varies from 6% in the community to 1.7% in the university setting. Possibly, these findings may be explained by the drug's wider use in the community. In our own setting, the vast majority of urinary strains of *Staphylococcus epidermidis* and *S. saprophyticus* have remained sensitive to nitrofurans. Resistance of *E. coli* to the fluoroquinolones was not seen when they were first intensively used. Recently, two resistant strains have been isolated in our laboratory (*vide infra*).

A survey of urinary isolate resistance patterns to commonly used antibiotics in one community in Britain indicated that nitrofurantoin and cephradine were more likely than other drugs to be active against *E. coli* and all other isolates studied (5). In evaluating the sensitivities of isolates from general practice patients, there appears to be little to differentiate ampicillin, trimethoprim, and sulfonamide. These antibiotics are active against only 60% to 80% of the strains tested, compared with 90% to 95% for nitrofurantoin. For perspective, hospital isolates were only slightly less susceptible than those from community patients (6).

For uncomplicated UTI, most physicians in Western Europe will administer empiric therapy without obtaining a culture. However, cultures and sensitivity tests are important in the management of recurrent UTIs, to differentiate relapse from reinfection and to select an appropriate antibiotic for ongoing therapy.

Table 3 Susceptibility of common uropathogens to selected antimicrobials

	N	Ampicillin			Amoxicillin plus clavulanic acid			Trimethoprim-sulfamethoxazole			Nitrofurantoin			Norfloxacin		
		R	I	S	R	I	S	R	I	S	R	I	S	R	I	S
Multicenter studies[a]																
Escherichia coli 1985	664	41	0.7	58.3	4		96	27.1	0.6	72.3	6	3.2	90.8	0	0.3	99.7
E. coli 1988	305				15.7	17.7	66.6									
Staphylococcus epidermidis	21	62	19	19	33		67				0		100	0		100
S. saprophyticus	12	8.4	41.6	50				25		75	0		100	0		100
St Luc University Hospital																
E. coli	1137	42	1	57	8	5	87	21	1	78	1.7	1	97.3	0.2	0	99.8
S. epidermidis	45	80		20	43		57	58	7	35	2.5		97.5	27.5	2.5	70
S. saprophyticus	17	29		71	14		86	29		71	0		100	6	6	88
Pseudomonas aeruginosa	84													7	5	88

Key: N = number of cases; R = resistant strains (%); I = intermediate strains (%); S = susceptible strains according to National Committee for Clinical Laboratory Standards.
[a](Data from references 6, 7, 8.)

For uncomplicated UTI, a high concentration of an active form of the antimicrobial should be obtained in the urine. High serum levels are desirable only in cases of parenchyma or bloodstream invasion. In the other instances, urinary specificity is a distinct advantage. Generalized action of the drug through high serum levels will tend to modify the commensal flora of the body cavities and invite superinfections (5).

It is important, therefore, when treating cystitis, to use an antibiotic with a low serum level so as not to disrupt the flora in other areas of the body. With optimal management of lower urinary tract infection (LUTI), the active drug is confined largely to the urine, so no changes are induced in the flora of the vagina or intestine. Thus, the development of troublesome yeast vaginitis can be minimized (9).

Recurrence of LUTI is common, because of the possibility of fecal flora invasion from the bowel reservoir. Constant investigational efforts are providing better understanding of its pathophysiology (10). Choosing an antibiotic that has no effect on the fecal flora is an important therapeutic goal, because such agents are not selective for resistant microorganisms and, therefore, minimize recurrent infection. Medications that alter bacteria in the bowel, either by poor absorption from the gastrointestinal (GI) tract or by high serum levels, are to be avoided (9).

SAFETY AND SIDE-EFFECTS OF ANTI-INFECTIVE AGENTS

Sulfonamides, TMP-SMX, trimethoprim

Simple sulfonamides are rarely used alone in Europe. Co-trimoxazole is, however, very popular, as is trimethoprim alone, which is as effective with fewer side-effects. GI disturbances and allergic reactions such as skin rashes may occur (11). Granulocytopenia, thrombocytopenia, and, rarely, agranulocytosis have been described (11). Macrocytic anemia due to folic acid deficiency may occur. Regular complete blood cell counts are recommended during prolonged therapy. In rare cases, neurotoxicity (psychosis, neuritis) and hepatic toxicity have been reported (11). TMP-SMX is contraindicated during pregnancy. When prescribed for women of child-bearing age, consideration should be given to evaluating the risk : benefit ratio. Another major problem is the emergence of resistance (27% of *E. coli* infections have become resistant to sulfonamides in our population, 38% in one English community) (3,6).

Nitrofurantoin

The nitrofurantoins are the most widely used antimicrobials in the treatment of UTIs in Belgium (Table 4) (11). They are rapidly eliminated in the urine,

Table 4 *Percentage of empiric prescriptions*

Nitrofurantoin	32.3
Quinolones	25.0
Trimethoprim-sulfamethoxazole	21.5
Ampicillin/amoxicillin	9.0
Cephalosporins	1.9
Others	10.3
TOTAL	100.0

(Data from reference 16.)

where they appear at high concentration in an active form. They have a wide activity spectrum including gram-positive and gram-negative organisms. Most *Proteus* sp are poorly sensitive and *Pseudomonas* is resistant. Nitrofurantoin does not affect fecal or vaginal flora. Despite prolonged usage in Europe, resistance to nitrofurantoin has not occurred to a significant extent (Table 3). There is no cross-resistance with other antibiotics.

The more common side effects associated with nitrofurantoin use are generally not serious. Nausea and gastric irritation can be a problem, depending upon the preparation (12). The usual daily dose of macrocrystalline forms is generally well tolerated. In exceptional cases, acute pulmonary reactions have been described; these require immediate discontinuation of therapy. Chronic pulmonary interstitial fibrosis has been described rarely, generally after prolonged therapy and especially in older patients. Peripheral neuropathy occurs rarely and is associated with treatment of patients with impaired renal function (12).

Ampicillin

Poorly absorbed from the GI tract, ampicillin gives rise to a high incidence of bowel flora modification with the risk of inducing resistance and superinfections. The commonly described incidence of *Candida* vaginitis is 25% (13). The widespread use of aminopenicillins has made a large proportion of enterobactericeae resistant (Table 3).

Amoxicillin

Absorption from the GI tract is better than that of ampicillin. In combination with a β-lactamase inhibitor (clavulanic acid) it retains a useful spectrum of activity. However, a mounting incidence of resistant strains has been reported in 1988 compared with that of 1985 (for *E. coli* 15.7% versus 5.8%) (7). In one community in Britain, the resistance of *E. coli* to ampicillin increased from 11% during 1975–77 to 32% during 1982–84 (5). The incidence of diarrhea and GI disturbance is higher than with amoxicillin alone. These compounds can be used during pregnancy. Other side-effects of both ampicillin and amoxicillin include skin rashes and the well known allergic reactions to penicillins with potential for anaphylactic reactions.

Nalidixic acid

Against most gram-negative uropathogens—not *Pseudomonas*—nalidixic acid is active. Resistance develops rapidly, especially if an inadequate dosage is used. High doses are therefore recommended. Side-effects, including nausea and vomiting, rash, and photosensitization are related to dosage. At high doses, central nervous system symptoms, such as dizziness, headaches, and convulsions, may occur.

Newer quinolones

Many analogs of nalidixic acid have been synthesized. Norfloxacin has been available in Western Europe for more than three years. Minimum inhibitory concentrations for most uropathogens are very low. Biologically, there is cross-resistance between the analogs of nalidixic acid, including the new quinolones. These compounds have such high activity, however, that resistant pathogens to nalidixic acid, although less sensitive to the new quinolones, are still well within their therapeutic range. However, the potential for development of resistance is an ever-present concern. In that respect, we have noted resistance of urinary *Pseudomonas aeruginosa* in our institution (7% resistant isolates plus 5% with intermediate sensitivity). Even some resistant *E. coli* have been found in the last few months, after prolonged usage and repeated treatment courses (6).

Fluoroquinolones are contraindicated in children, pregnant females, and epileptics. If prescribed to women of child-bearing age, a determination of pregnancy should be made. Typical side-effects include nausea and vomiting, anorexia, gastric distress, and diarrhea. Dizziness and headaches have also been described; however, rashes are rare. At the usual dosage recommended for uncomplicated UTIs (400 mg b.i.d), side-effects are uncommon (4%). However, the cost of the new quinolones is quite high.

Oral cephalosporins

Not active against enterococci, the oral cephalosporins (cephalexin, cefradine, cefaclor, and cefadroxyl) often retain activity against bacteria resistant to ampicillin. They are useful as second choice drugs for allergic patients or during pregnancy, but are relatively expensive.

Duration of therapy

Optimal duration of therapy for uncomplicated UTI remains controversial. Some authors recommend single-dose therapy, claiming an adequate response rate and the additional advantage of making a differential diagnosis of complicated UTI in case of failure of the single dose treatment. It is, however, our impression that clinical response rates are not as high, and recurrence is somewhat greater compared with a longer course of treatment. We recommend up to a seven-day course of medication in cases of first infection, and seven- to 14-day treatment for recurrent uncomplicated infections of the lower urinary tract. This corresponds to the common attitude practiced in Belgium, as illustrated by a recent study. Single-dose treatment was only rarely prescribed; an equal proportion of treatment had been prescribed with and without culture and sensitivity results, except for long-term treatment, where sensitivity results were more frequently obtained (14).

CRITERIA FOR SELECTING THERAPY IN UNCOMPLICATED UTI

The selection of an antimicrobial for treatment of UTI depends on:

- Severity of the infection
- Prevalence of the usual uropathogens and their potential sensitivity
- Expected compliance of the patient, which is a function of the ease of administration, side-effects, and total cost.

Uncomplicated UTI includes asymptomatic bacteriuria, acute cystitis, and acute pyelonephritis.

Symptomatic cystitis in women is by far the most common problem with *E. coli* the most prevalent infective organism. Many drugs are available to treat these infections, and selection is made primarily on the expected susceptibility of the organism, cost, and toxicity.

Achieving high urine concentration is not a practical problem, as most available oral antimicrobials reach very high concentrations in the urine. This explains their clinical efficacy despite *in vitro* resistance of the causative organism.

Frequency of recurrence is the major problem associated with uncomplicated UTI. Selection of an agent which does not easily induce bacterial resistance is important.

Most uropathogens originate from the bowel flora. Therefore, selection of a drug that is promptly absorbed from the GI tract and does not appear in the large bowel, will leave the fecal flora intact and will prevent clinical resistance.

The duration of therapy for uncomplicated UTI should be proportional to the probability of invasion of urinary parenchyma. In a superficial infection, shorter courses are indicated. I have settled on a three- to 10-day regimen because of the difficulty of diagnosing tissue invasion and the unpredictability of patient response. For low-dose, long-term therapy, a drug that does not affect bowel and vaginal flora is essential.

In Europe, the following medications are usually recommended in uncomplicated UTI: nitrofurantoin macrocrystals; TMP-SMX, or trimethoprim alone; amoxicillin alone or, preferably, in combination with clavulanic acid, and, in reserve, the new quinolones. The resistance of *E. coli* to ampicillin (45%), to amoxicillin-clavulanic acid (15%), and to TMP-SMX (22%) is becoming a real clinical problem (8).

In Belgium, nitrofurantoin macrocrystals remains one of the first choices (Table 4). Most common urinary pathogens remain sensitive, including *E. coli* and *S. saprophyticus*; and the drug is inexpensive, safe, and available in a convenient package for ease in administration and compliance.

Although their costs are high, quinolones are widely used and very effective. However, resistance with nosocomial organisms, as well as with some of the common urinary pathogens after repeated courses of therapy and prolonged usage, is appearing. Because of their unknown potential for resistance and cost, in our opinion, the new quinolones should be restricted to complicated UTIs or pathogens resistant to simple, classic antibiotics.

REFERENCES

(1) EEC: *Comparative tables of the Social Security schemes in the member states of the European communities*. 14th ed. ECSC-EEC Brussels, Luxembourg 1988.
(2) Infections non compliquées de l'appareil urinaire inférieur chez la femme non enciente. Aspect statistique: envoi chez le spécialiste. *IMS Bull d'Informations Méd Statist* 1986; **34**: 16.
(3) Gaymans R, Haverkorn MJ, Valkenburg HA, Goslings WR. A prospective study of urinary-tract infections in a Dutch general practice. *Lancet* 1976; **ii**: 674–677.
(4) Pedler SJ, Bint AJ. Management of bacteriuria in pregnancy. *Drugs* 1987; **33**: 413–421.
(5) Brumfitt W, Hamilton-Miller JMT. Bacterial resistance: how to keep it in check. *Recent advances in treatment of urinary tract infections*. Proceedings of symposium. Amsterdam: Norwich Eaton. Sept. 18, 1985.
(6) St Luc University Hospital (Brussels), microbiology department: Preliminary findings, 1986–1988.
(7) Verbist L: A Belgian multicentre *in vitro* study of norfloxacin. *J Antimicrob Chemother* 1988; **22** (suppl C): 35–43.
(8) Verbist L. Belgian multicenter *in vitro* study of norfloxacin. *Acta Clin Belg* 1985; **40**: 167–173.
(9) Parsons CL. Antibiotic selection for lower urinary tract infections. *Fam Pract Recert* 1987; **9** (suppl 2): 9.

(10) Kunin CM. Urinary tract infection: new information concerning pathogenesis and management. *J Urol* 1982; **128**: 1233.
(11) Van Cangh PJ. Quand faut-il aller plus loin? *IMS Bull d'Informations Méd Statist* 1982; **34**: 13.
(12) Sanford JP. *Guide to antimicrobial therapy*. West Bethesda, Md.: Antimicrobials Therapy, 1988.
(13) Parsons CL. Lower urinary tract infections in women. *Urol Clin North Am* 1987; **14**: 247–250.
(14) Crokaert F, Yourassowski E. Traitement des infections urinaires par dose unique d'antibiotiques. *IMS Bull d'Informations Méd Statist* 1986; **35**: 14.
(15) Ministry of Public Health, Belgium: Répertoire commenté des médicaments, 1987.
(16) Verbist L. Infections non compliquées de l'appareil urinaire inférieur chez la femme non enceinte: aspect médical. *IMS Bull d'Informations Méd Statist* 1986: 35.

An open-label randomized comparative trial of nitrofurantoin macrocrystals and TMP-SMX in acute urinary tract infection in Colombia

E. Gomez

National University of Colombia School of Medicine Bogotá, Colombia

ABSTRACT

A study to compare the efficacy and tolerance of nitrofurantoin macrocrystals[a] with trimethoprim-sulfamethoxazole (TMP-SMX)[b] in the treatment of acute uncomplicated urinary tract infections was performed at the San Juan de Dios Hospital in Bogotá, Colombia, from June 1986 to January 1988. The study involved nonpregnant women and was an open parallel, randomized, prospective trial.

Twenty-six women received nitrofurantoin macrocrystals, 100 mg, q.i.d., and 24 women received trimethoprim, 160 mg, and sulfamethoxazole, 800 mg, b.i.d., for 10 days. At the time of entry, the two groups were comparable as to signs, symptoms, and the results of laboratory urine tests and cultures.

Response to treatment was rated on the basis of the clinical evaluation, disappearance of signs and symptoms, and urine tests and cultures performed on days 3, 11, and 18 to 19 after the start of treatment. *In vitro* susceptibility rates of the strains isolated in the patients who completed the study were 50 of 53 (94.34%) and 41 of 53 (77.36%) for nitrofurantoin macrocrystals and TMP-SMX, respectively ($p<0.05$). In 24 of 26 (92.3%) of the patients treated with nitrofurantoin macrocrystals, and in 19 (79.17%) of the 24 patients treated with TMP-SMX, the treatment provided both a clinical and a bacteriologic cure ($p=0.24$). Two of the patients treated with nitrofurantoin macrocrystals (7.7%) and five (20.8%) of those who received TMP-SMX were considered bacteriologic treatment failures. Taking into account its specificity for the urinary tract, nitrofurantoin macrocrystals can be considered the drug of first choice for effective management of cystitis.

INTRODUCTION

Women have more than twice as many urinary tract infections (UTIs) as men, and 70% of their infections occur between the ages of 20 and 54 years (Table 1) (1).

---

[a]Macrodantin® capsulas (nitrofurantoin macrocrystals capsules, 50 mg). Norwich Colombiana, SA.
[b]Bactrim® comprimidos (trimethoprim, 80 mg, and sulfamethoxazole, 400 mg). Roche SA, Colombia.

Management of urinary tract infections, edited by Lloyd H. Harrison, 1990; Royal Society of Medicine Services International Congress and Symposium Series No. 154, published by Royal Society of Medicine Services Limited.

Table 1 Demographics of patients who have UTI

Characteristic	%
Age (years)	
0–19	19.8
20–54	70.2
55 and older	10.0
Sex	
Males	30.1
Females	69.9

Source: Indice Nacional de Terapeutica y Enfermedades (INTE). Diagnostica 59, Infeccion Uniaria, June 1988.

Table 2 Microorganisms isolated according to treatment groups

	Nitrofurantoin macrocrystals	TMP-SMX
Total patients	26	24
Total microorganisms	26	27
Escherichia coli	24	20
Klebsiella oxytoca	—	3
Klebsiella sp	1	1
Proteus mirabilis	1	1
P. vulgaris	—	1
Alcaligenes faecalis	—	1

Cystitis is the UTI physicians see most often. Seventy-four percent of the time it is uncomplicated by other disease. *Escherichia coli* is the predominant uropathogen in uncomplicated UTIs (Table 2) (2).

The essential guidelines for choosing a drug to treat an acute, uncomplicated UTI must include efficacy, safety, and specificity for the urinary tract, as evidenced by low serum and high urinary levels, ability to spare the normal flora, low toxicity, and acceptable cost (3). The scope of the treatment must be sufficiently wide to cover the majority of pathogens suspected of causing the infection, based on the infection site and the type of host (4).

The ideal antibacterial agent must have the following characteristics:
- Convenient oral administration
- A wide spectrum of antimicrobial activity against the most common uropathogens—*E. coli, Klebsiella,* and enterococcus—with low serum and high urinary levels
- Low vaginal concentration, so the normal vaginal flora will be undisturbed
- Urinary tract specificity to preserve the intestinal flora without promoting proliferation of resistant organisms and fungi
- Minimal undesirable side effects
- Low cost.

COLOMBIAN PATIENT PROFILE

Schooling level has an impact on patient compliance, as it correlates with the patient's ability to understand instructions. In Colombia, only 75.1% of the total population is literate (5). The per capita daily earnings average $5.31 in US dollars (6).

Because pharmacy sellers do not always insist on proof of prescription, Colombian patients tend to self-medicate. The result is indiscriminate use of antimicrobial drugs. Such self-medication leads to resistance, as well as underdosage, deficient identification of the causative organism, and failure to determine the organism's susceptibility.

This study was designed to compare the efficacy and safety of nitrofurantoin macrocrystals (Macrodantin®) and TMP-SMX in the treatment of acute uncomplicated UTIs. Both drugs are available and commonly used in Colombia, as well as elsewhere in the Latin American market, to treat UTIs.

MATERIALS AND METHODS

A randomized, prospective study of outpatient women between the ages of 18 and 60 was conducted at the San Juan de Dios Hospital from June 1, 1986 to January 31, 1988. All patients had one or more of the following symptoms within the five days prior to the trial enrollment: dysuria, frequency, burning, pyuria, and hematuria (Table 3).

The following types of patients were excluded from the study:
- Women whose pretreatment uroculture failed to demonstrate colonies of *E. coli* greater than 10^5/ml or colonies of other uropathogens greater than 10^4/ml.
- Women who experienced one or more UTIs within six months prior to the study enrollment
- Women whose symptoms included high temperature, lumbar pain, urethral secretions, and/or vaginal discharge
- Women suspected of having sexually transmitted disease
- Women who had taken antibiotics within the five days before enrollment.

Other conditions for exclusion were: allergy to the drugs under study, any major surgery during the previous six months, glucose-6-phosphate dehydrogenase

Table 3 *Characteristics of study population*

	Nitrofurantoin macrocrystals ($n=26$)		TMP-SMX ($n=24$)		
	Mean	SD	Mean	SD	p^a
Age (years)	43	12	35	11	0.25
Days for evolution of signs and symptoms	3.6	1.5	4.2	1.28	0.2
Weight (kg)	59	9	57	10	0.45
Signs and symptoms at entry	n		n		p^b
Burning	24		21		0.66
Frequency	23		22		0.92
Dysuria	22		21		0.91
Pyuria	20		17		0.87
Hematuria	7		4		0.50

^{a}Two-sample t test; ^{b}Fisher exact test (two-tail)
Key: TMP-SMX = trimethoprim-sulfamethoxazole; n = number of patients; SD = standard deviation; p = probability; kg = kilograms

deficiency, renal or hepatic insufficiency, a history of urinary lithiasis or of morphologic anomalies of the urinary tract, and pregnancy.

Patients entering the study were randomly assigned to receive a 10-day course of one of the following treatments: nitrofurantoin macrocrystals, 50 mg×2, q.i.d., or trimethoprim, 80 mg, and sulfamethoxazole, 400 mg×2, b.i.d. Treatment was begun on day 1. On days 3 (visit 2), 11 (visit 3), and 18–19 (visit 4), the symptoms recorded at entry were reassessed and urine samples were obtained for microscopic examination and culture. Response to treatment was rated on the basis of bacteriologic results as follows: cure, improvement, no effectiveness, cure with relapse, and cure with reinfection.

The following guidelines were used to assess results:

Cure. If the causative organism was eradicated or considerably decreased (colonies ≤ 1000/ml) on visit 2, with the same pattern maintained at visits 3 and 4.

Improvement. If at visit 2 or 3 the original causative organism was present in the urine in colony counts of greater than 1000 but $\leq 10^5$/ml for *E. coli* or $\leq 10^4$/ml for other uropathogens.

Failure

Cure with relapse: If the causative organism was eradicated or drastically reduced in the culture count (colonies fewer than 1000/ml) at follow-up visits 2 and 3, but colonies of the same organism were found in the urine in concentrations greater than 10^5/ml for *E. coli* or greater than 10^4/ml for other uropathogens at visit 4. (Possible relapse if the colony counts were less than previously mentioned.)

Cure with reinfection: If the original causative organism was eradicated or drastically reduced in colony counts at visits 2 and 3, but a different organism was found in the urine in concentrations greater than 10^5/ml for *E. coli* or greater than 10^4/ml for other urinary pathogens at visit 4, a reinfection had occurred following a cure. (Possible reinfection if the colony counts were less than previously mentioned.)

Ineffective: If at visits 2 or 3 the original causative organism was present in the urine in colony counts of greater than 10^5/ml for *E. coli* or more than 10^4/ml for other urinary pathogens.

Clinical evaluation of how effectively treatment controlled the signs and symptoms was based on the number of each present at the first visit and at every follow-up visit.

Treatment failure was also considered to have occurred when one or more of the symptoms observed after admission to the study had worsened at visit 2, or when adverse side effects or untoward reactions were ascribable to treatment and required its discontinuation.

STATISTICAL METHODS

The Wilcoxon two-sample t test and the Fisher exact test were used to compare the characteristics of study population and signs and symptoms present at admission and to compare the efficacy of the two treatments. McNemar's method was used to compare proportions in susceptibility frequencies.

RESULTS

The study involved 56 women, six of whom were excluded from analysis for failing to meet the inclusion criteria. Of the 50 patients assessed, 26 received nitrofurantoin macrocrystals and 24 received TMP-SMX. The groups were comparable as to demographics, history, and signs and symptoms present at admission. *Escherichia coli* was the pathogen most frequently isolated; it was found in 92.3% of the patients who received nitrofurantoin macrocrystals, and in 83.3% of those who received TMP-SMX.

Fifty of the 53 strains isolated in the patients who completed the study were susceptible to nitrofurantoin macrocrystals, and 41 of 53 (77.36%) were susceptible to TMP-SMX ($p<0.05$). The resistant strains isolated in the nitrofurantoin macrocrystals group were *Klebsiella oxytoca*. All but one (*Klebsiella* sp) of the resistant strains isolated in the TMP-SMX group were *E. coli*. All of the *E. coli* strains isolated in the patients who completed the study were susceptible to nitrofurantion macrocrystals, and 33 of 44 (75%) were susceptible to TMP-SMX ($p<0.05$).

The clinical effectiveness for each patient was indicated by the decrease from day 1 in the number of signs and symptoms as determined on days 3, 11, and 18. The mean changes between the treatment groups at subsequent visits were compared (Table 4). The improvements in numbers, or scores, of signs and symptoms through the follow-up between the treatment groups were not significantly different. The overall bacteriologic cure and failure rates for the two drugs are shown in Table 5. All patients who achieved a bacteriologic cure were free of signs and symptoms by the end of therapy and during follow-up. No patients experienced worsening of signs and symptoms despite achieving bacteriologic improvement or cure. Thus, in 24 of 26 (92.3%) patients treated with nitrofurantoin macrocrystals and in 19 of 24 (79.17%) patients treated with TMP-SMX, the treatment provided both clinical and bacteriologic cure ($p=0.24$). In two of 26 (7.69%) patients who received nitrofurantoin macrocrystals and in three of 24 who received TMP-SMX, the treatment was not effective. Also two of 24 (8.33%) patients who received TMP-SMX had cure with relapse.

Three of the total patient population who completed the study had a bacterial strain resistant to nitrofurantoin macrocrystals. One person, from whom *Proteus mirabilis* was isolated, was randomly assigned to receive nitrofurantoin macrocrystals and subsequently had both clinical and bacteriologic cure.

Table 4 *Mean number of signs and symptoms (score) from each visit and change from baseline (day 1)*

Visit/day	Nitrofurantoin macrocrystals Score[a]	Changes[b]	n	TMP-SMX Score[a]	Changes[b]	n	p[c]
Baseline (1)	4.92	0	26	4.92	0	24	0.84
2/3	0.69	−4.23	26	0.40	−4.52	23	0.23
3/11	0.23	−4.69	26	0.63	−4.29	24	0.51
4/18	0.04	−4.88	25	0.40	−4.52	23	0.44

[a]For each visit the score was calculated by dividing the total number of signs and symptoms present at that visit by the number of evaluable patients for that visit. [b]Each score for a specified visit was subtracted from the baseline (day 1) score, and these differences appear in the table. [c]Wilcoxon two-sample test used for the two treatment groups.
Key: TMP-SMX=trimethoprim-sulfamethoxazole; n=number of patients; p=probability.

Table 5 *Nitrofurantoin macrocrystals vs TMP-SMX: outcome of treatment*

	Nitrofurantoin macrocrystals n	Nitrofurantoin macrocrystals %	TMP-SMX n	TMP-SMX %	Total n	Total %
Total population	28	—	28	—	56	—
Exclusions[a]	2	7.14	4	14.29	6	10.71
Patients assessed	26	—	24	—	50	—
Cure[b]	24	92.30	19	79.17	43	86
Failure	2	7.69	5	20.83	7	14
Ineffective	2	7.69	3	12.50	5	10
Cure with relapse	—	—	2	8.33	2	4
Cure with reinfection	—	—	—	—	—	—

[a]*Failed to meet inclusion criteria.* [b]*Cure vs failure* $p=0.24$; *the Fisher exact test (two-tail) was used.*
Key: TMP-SMX = trimethoprim sulfamethoxazole; n = number of patients.

Twelve of the total patient population who completed the study had a bacterial strain resistant to TMP-SMX, and only two—both *E. coli* isolates—were randomly assigned to the drug. One of these patients had both clinical and bacteriologic cure; in the other, treatment was ineffective. This imbalanced distribution occurred by chance according to random allocation. Both drugs were well tolerated by the study population and produced no apparent adverse reactions.

DISCUSSION

In this study, nitrofurantoin macrocrystals was shown to be significantly better *in vitro* than was TMP-SMX, which frequently develops bacterial resistance (7). In this sample, the overall success rate for nitrofurantoin macrocrystals was superior to that for TMP-SMX in the treatment of acute uncomplicated UTI. The difference, however, was not statistically significant.

According to the random allocation, patients with 10 of 12 of the strains resistant to TMP-SMX were allocated to receive nitrofurantoin macrocrystals. Although the unbalanced distribution occurred by chance, being favorable to TMP-SMX, it may have influenced the final TMP-SMX cure rate obtained in this trial. Therefore, some speculation can be made about the possibility of lesser cure rates for TMP-SMX in a more balanced distribution.

UTIs, more common in women than in men, are usually caused by pathogenic agents in the periurethral or intestinal flora. Drugs that modify flora must be used judiciously to not risk generating needless bacterial resistance. They must cover the majority of pathogens suspected of causing the infection and preserve the intestinal flora without promoting proliferation of other organisms such as fungi. This ideal antibacterial agent should produce minimal undesirable side effects and be easy to administer. Finally, low cost is an important factor to consider.

On the basis of the data reported in this study and on broad experience with the drug all over the world, we propose that nitrofurantoin macrocrystals meets the requirements for consideration as the bactericidal agent of choice for treating acute uncomplicated UTIs.

REFERENCES

(1) *Indice Nacional de Terapeutica y Enfermedades* (INTE), Diagnostica 59, Infeccion Uniaria. June 1988.
(2) Parsons CL, Lacey SS. Urinary tract infections. In: Buchsbaum HJ, Schmidt JD, eds. *Gynecologic and obstetric urology*, 2nd ed. Philadelphia: WB Saunders Co, 1982: 347-372, chap 24.
(3) Parsons CL. Antibiotic selection for treatment of lower urinary tract infections. *Fam Pract Recert* 1987; **9** (2): 9.
(4) Hanno P. Etiology of cystitis; factors affecting its management strategies. *Fam Pract Recert* 1987; **9** (2): 14.
(5) *Colombia Estadistica*. Departmento Administrativo Nacional de Estadistica (DANE), Colombia. 1985: 163.
(6) *Colombia Estadistica*. Departmento Administrativo Nacional de Estadistica (DANE), Colombia. 1988: 397.
(7) Wilkowske CJ, Hermans PE. General principles of antimicrobial therapy. *Mayo Clin Proc* 1987; **62**: 789-798.

Inhibition of bacterial protein synthesis by nitrofurantoin macrocrystals: An explanation for the continued efficacy of nitrofurantoin

C. C. McOsker, J. R. Pollack and J. A. Andersen

Norwich Eaton Pharmaceuticals, Inc., Norwich, New York, USA

ABSTRACT

Thirty years after the introduction of nitrofuran antimicrobials, development of clinical resistance to nitrofurantoin (Macrodantin®) macrocrystals among strains of susceptible species is almost nonexistent. In contrast, significant resistance to all other classes of antimicrobials has emerged within a short time after they were placed into widespread use. To determine the cause of this phenomenon, we studied the mechanism of action of nitrofurantoin macrocrystals with the specific aim of defining their intracellular target. Our analysis indicated nitrofurantoin inhibits protein synthesis at the level of the ribosome, acting through the formation of active intermediates, which can form covalent bonds with ribosomal proteins. The data further indicate these intermediates bind nonspecifically to almost every ribosomal protein. This suggests a reason for absence of resistance.

Simultaneous mutation of almost all ribosomal proteins would be required to avoid inhibition of protein synthesis by nitrofurantoin intermediates, a highly unlikely occurrence. Furthermore, if mutations occurred on such a sweeping scale, they would likely be lethal to the bacteria. These conclusions suggest that the continued use of nitrofurantoin macrocrystals as the first-line therapy for management of acute and recurrent urinary tract infections is unlikely to lead to any demonstrable development of resistance among initially susceptible pathogens.

INTRODUCTION

Over the past 50 years, enormous effort has gone into finding means to kill or inhibit the growth of pathogenic bacteria. This effort has resulted in the isolation and screening of thousands of new compounds that act through diverse mechanisms, not all of which are well understood. As a result of this intensive research and development, an array of new antibiotics is continually being made available for clinical use. The introduction and use of each new antibacterial agent has almost invariably been followed by the development of strains of bacteria resistant to its action, leading to a quest for still more powerful antimicrobials.

Management of urinary tract infections, edited by Lloyd H. Harrison, 1990; Royal Society of Medicine Services International Congress and Symposium Series No. 154, published by Royal Society of Medicine Services Limited.

The relationship between the development of new antimicrobials and the appearance of resistant strains can be seen most clearly in the case of β-lactam antibiotics, which primarily interfere with bacterial cell wall synthesis. The most widespread form of resistance to these agents is caused by the synthesis of enzymes (β-lactamases) that degrade the antibiotic. Gram-negative bacteria such as *Escherichia coli* demonstrate widespread and increasing resistance of this type to ampicillin, amoxicillin, and other older β-lactams, as well as the newer β-lactams such as cephalosporins (1). Significant resistance can also result from alteration of the target proteins to which the β-lactams must bind to be effective (2).

Resistance to antimicrobials such as the sulfonamides (1), which act by inhibiting crucial metabolic steps, also occurs frequently. One strategy to reduce the rate at which resistance develops has been to combine two different agents, such as trimethoprim and sulfamethoxazole (TMP-SMX). However, the rate of resistance to this combination, although lower than to either agent alone, has recently been increasing, significantly limiting the drug's overall clinical activity (3-6).

Resistance can develop rapidly; for example, resistance to fluoroquinolones such as norfloxacin (Noroxin®) and ciprofloxacin (Cipro®) has already been observed in clinical situations, even though these drugs have been introduced only within the past five years (7,8). Generally, however, the degree of resistance to a particular antibiotic is strongly correlated with both the length of time since introduction and its frequency of use. An interesting exception is nitrofurantoin (Macrodantin®) macrocrystals. Nitrofurantoin is highly active against common urinary tract pathogens and is bactericidal at levels achieved in the urinary tract. Although nitrofurantoin has been in broad clinical use for almost 30 years, bacteria within its spectrum remain almost uniformly susceptible, and significant clinical resistance has not been observed (9). Over the same period, the predominant pathogens in UTIs, *E. coli* and *Staphylococcus saprophyticus*, have developed widespread resistance to other antimicrobial agents (10).

At least part of the antibacterial activity of nitrofuran antimicrobials is due to inhibition of protein synthesis at the level of the bacterial ribosome. The antimicrobial effect appears to be caused by the formation of reactive intermediates by enzymatic reduction within the bacterial cell (9,11). A study was undertaken to determine the mechanism by which nitrofurantoin macrocrystals exerted this antibacterial activity. Results suggest that both the mode of action and intracellular targets of nitrofurantoin are distinct from other antibiotic classes, and these differences may account for the lack of resistance development in clinical experience.

RESULTS

Previous studies (9) showed that nitrofuran antimicrobials, such as nitrofurazone, underwent enzymatic reduction within bacteria, resulting in the formation of highly reactive intermediates. The probable pathways of nitrofuran reduction to produce reactive intermediates are shown in Fig. 1. It should first be noted that the antibacterial effects of nitrofurantoin (and other nitrofurans) appear to be due to the nitro moiety (Fig. 1). Briefly, initial metabolic steps appear to involve initial reduction to either of two reactive species (1 or 2), followed by subsequent reduction to another reactive species (3), followed by reduction to a fourth (4). The initial three products (1 to 3) have not been isolated; all are highly reactive

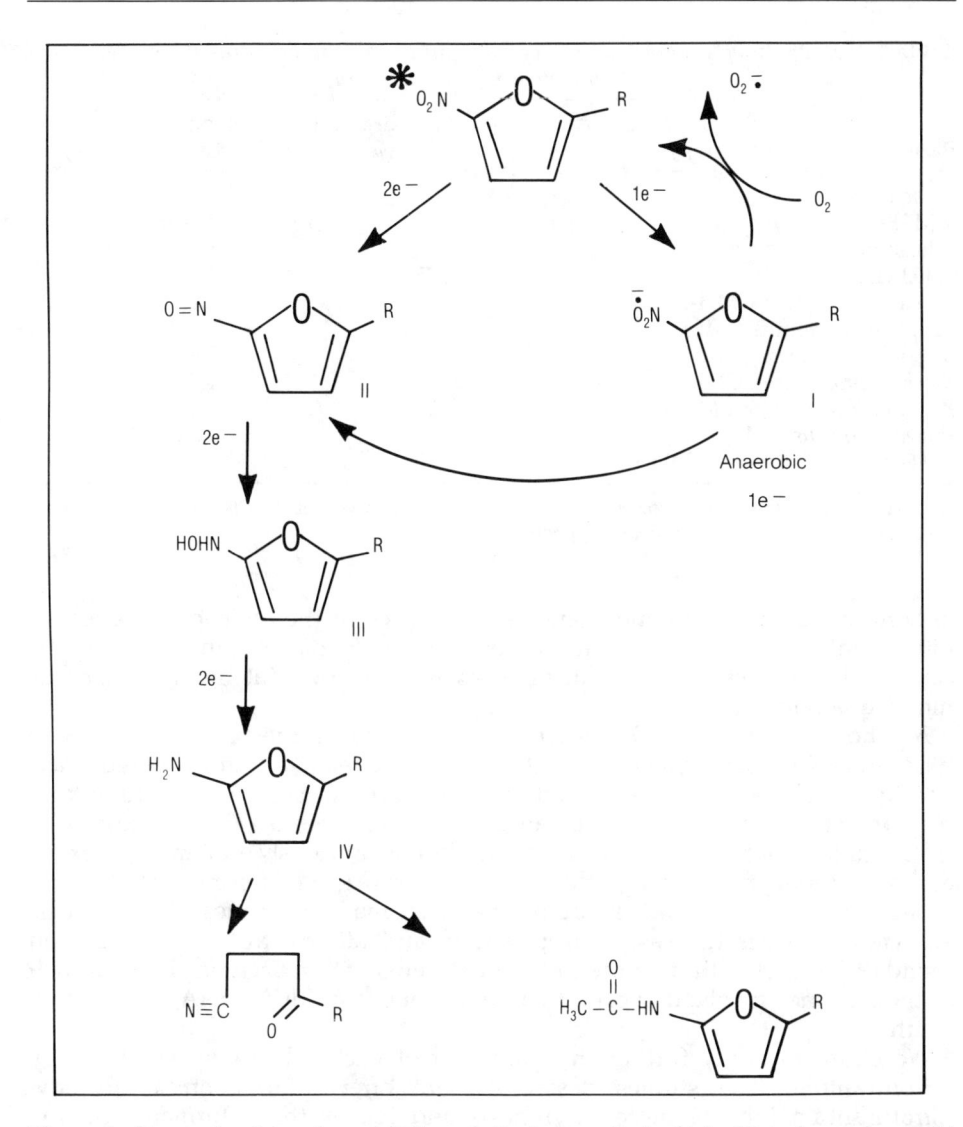

Figure 1 *Proposed pathway for metabolism of nitrofuran antimicrobials. (Data from reference 9.)*

species, and their presence has been inferred from either the final metabolic products observed or from spectroscopic observations.

These reactive intermediates are electrophilic and therefore able to undergo covalent reaction with the nucleophilic groups which are widely distributed on proteins and nucleic acids within the bacterial cell. In the present study, representatives of common urinary tract pathogens were tested both for their nitrofurantoin sensitivity and for the amount of nitrofuran reductase activity present. Organisms tested were both nitrofurantoin susceptible (*E. coli, Enterobacter cloacae, Streptococcus faecalis, Staphylococcus aureus, S. epidermidis, S. saprophyticus*) and nonsusceptible (*Klebsiella pneumoniae, Proteus mirabilis* and *Pseudomonas aeruginosa*). Three strains of *E. coli* were included in this study: two (MRE600 and EC3669) were susceptible to nitrofurantoin, while the third (153R103) is not a clinical isolate but was made resistant to nitrofurantoin by

Table 1 *Sensitivity of urinary tract pathogens to nitrofurantoin macrocrystals correlates with nitrofurantoin reductase activity*

Bacteria	Nitrofurantoin MIC (μg/ml)	Reductase specific activity (mU/mg)[a]
Escherichia coli		
MRE600[b]	16	7.1
EC3669[b]	16	7.8
153R103[c]	250	2.1
Enterobacter cloacae CMH-9	32	9.2
Streptococcus faecalis CMH-6	16	6.6
Staphylococcus epidermidis CMH-7	8	7.8
Staph. saprophyticus CMH-6	8	4.5
Klebsiella pneumoniae CMH-2	128	2.1
Proteus mirabilis CMH-2	128	<0.3
Pseudomonas aeruginosa CMH-3	>128	<0.3

[a]1 U—1 μmol nitrofurantoin reduced per minute; [b]wild-type; [c]derived from EC-3669 by nitrosoguanidine mutagenesis. MIC=minimum inhibitory concentration.

in vitro nitrosoquanidine mutagenesis. Resistance to the antibacterial effect of nitrofurantoin, while not generally observed in *E. coli* in clinical situations, can be obtained by random mutagenesis with a powerful mutagen such as nitrosoquanidine.

As shown in Table 1, the degree of sensitivity of the bacterial strains to nitrofurantoin macrocrystals correlates with their relative nitrofuran reductase activity. Much less reductase activity was observed in both the nitrofurantoin-resistant strain of *E. coli* and in nonsusceptible bacteria. This suggests that nitrofurantoin macrocrystals, like other nitrofurans previously examined (9), exerts an antibacterial effect through the production of reactive intermediates that are capable of binding to and disrupting bacterial macromolecules. As would be expected if this is the case, nitrofurantoin and other nitrofurans have been found (9) to react with multiple sites and systems within bacteria (Table 2) such as the enzymes involved in carbohydrate metabolism, RNA, DNA, and protein synthesis.

We chose to study further the inhibition of bacterial protein synthesis by nitrofurantoin. The studies described here offer information as to how nitrofurantoin inhibits protein synthesis and relates this information to the potential for bacterial resistance development to nitrofurantoin.

Initial steps to identify potential bacterial sites of nitrofurantoin attack confirmed that treatment with nitrofurantoin macrocrystals inhibited protein synthesis. The rate of synthesis was determined by measuring the incorporation of the amino acid proline labeled with radioactive carbon (^{14}C) into proteins. A nitrofurantoin concentration of 20 μg/ml had no effect on protein synthesis, while 80 μg/ml

Table 2 *Sites of action of nitrofurantoin metabolites within bacteria*

- Carbohydrate metabolism
- RNA
- DNA
- Protein synthesis

Table 3 *Inhibition of protein synthesis by nitrofurantoin macrocrystals is due to an effect on the ribosome*

	Protein synthesis (% of control)[a]	
	Untreated ribosomes	Treated ribosomes
Treated accessory proteins	100	ND[b]
Untreated accessory proteins	100	45.2

E. coli MRE600 was incubated with nitrofurantoin macrocrystals (160 µg/ml) or with normal medium. Accessory proteins and ribosomal fractions were separated by ultracentrifugation and recombined in a cell-free protein synthesis system.

[a]Untreated ribosomes and untreated accessory proteins; [b]not determined.

produced transient inhibition, and 160 µg/ml produced essentially complete inhibition of protein synthesis. Although these concentrations are greater than the minimum inhibitory concentration (MIC) for nitrofurantoin against *E. coli*, high cell densities (approximately 1000-fold higher than normally seen in UTIs) were used. This, in turn, required the use of greater-than-normal concentrations of nitrofurantoin; these high drug concentrations do not indicate bacterial resistance. To determine the site of action for inhibition of protein synthesis by nitrofurantoin macrocrystals, bacteria were incubated either with or without 160 µg/ml of nitrofurantoin. Ribosomes and the accessory protein fraction which contains soluble enzymes necessary for protein synthesis were isolated from both bacterial populations by differential centrifugation. Nitrofurantoin-treated ribosomes were combined with untreated accessory proteins in a cell-free protein translation system and vice versa. The combination of nitrofurantoin-treated accessory proteins with untreated ribosomes gave a rate of protein synthesis equal to the control (both untreated). However, the combination of treated ribosomes and untreated accessory proteins resulted in 54.8% inhibition of protein synthesis (Table 3), indicating the ribosomes, and not the accessory proteins, are the primary target for nitrofurantoin inhibition of protein synthesis.

We then proceeded to define specifically which of the ribosomal proteins were attacked by the reactive nitrofurantoin intermediates. To determine this, *E. coli* were incubated with ^{14}C-labeled nitrofurantoin macrocrystals at a concentration of either 20, 80 or 160 µg/ml. Ribosomes were collected from these bacteria, and ribosomal proteins were solubilized and subjected to two-dimensional gel electrophoresis, which, as used here, separates ribosomal proteins by differences in charge/mass ratio at two different pHs (12). The resulting 'grid' is capable of cleanly resolving 43 of the 55 ribosomal proteins. The gels were stained with Coomassie blue to display separated proteins (Fig. 2). Each protein spot was then cut out of the gel, and the amount of radioactive label incorporated into each protein was determined by scintillation counting.

As Table 4 shows, almost every ribosomal protein is labeled with ^{14}C-nitrofurantoin at all three concentrations tested. This indicates that all (or almost all) ribosomal proteins are targets for the reactive nitrofurantoin intermediates. The relative percentage of label associated with each ribosomal protein under the three experimental conditions is shown in Fig. 3. A relatively nonspecific distribution of label is seen when bacteria are incubated either with 20, 80, or 160 µg/ml of nitrofurantoin macrocrystals. However, the total amount of labeled nitrofurantoin bound to ribosomal proteins increases severalfold with increasing concentration (data not shown), probably accounting for the inhibition of bacterial protein synthesis seen at higher concentrations of nitrofurantoin. In other words,

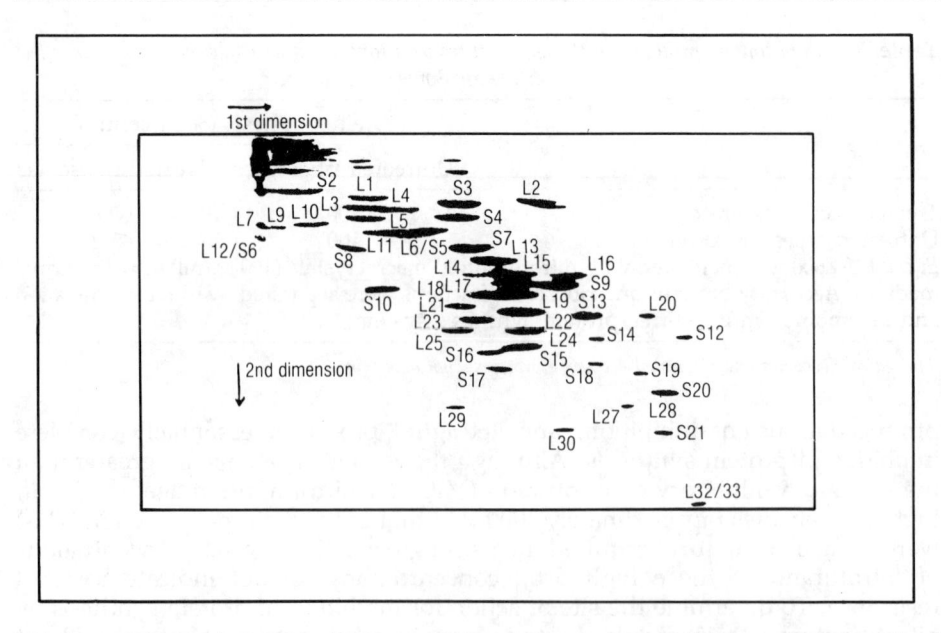

Figure 2 *Ribosomal proteins (300 μg total protein) were separated by two-dimensional gel electrophoresis as described by Geyl (12) (origin at upper left). Separated proteins were visualized by staining with Coomassie blue.*

Table 4 *Labeling of ribosomal proteins by varying concentrations of ^{14}C-nitrofurantoin*

	Number of proteins labeled[a]		
	20 μg/ml	80 μg/ml	160 μg/ml
No label detectable	1	0	0
<5% of total label	40	41	39
5%–10% of total label	2	2	24
>10% of total label	0	0	0

[a]Bacteria were incubated with nitrofurantoin for 45 min at 37°C, then ribosomal proteins were separated by two-dimensional gel electrophoresis and radioactivity in each protein determined.

it is the total *amount* of nitrofurantoin bound to the ribosome, and not interactions with specific sites, that accounts for inhibition of protein synthesis.

To further substantiate that nitrofurantoin-derived inhibition of protein synthesis was the result of binding of reactive intermediates to ribosomes and not due to another, undefined mechanism, bacteria were simultaneously incubated with nitrofurantoin and 2-mercaptoethanol (2-ME). The latter compound in excess would be expected to competitively bind to any reactive nitrofurantoin intermediates produced, thereby preventing attack on ribosomal proteins. As illustrated in Table 5, 2-ME restored the ability of *E. coli* to synthesize protein to the same extent to which it decreased the binding of radioactively labeled nitrofurantoin to the ribosome, suggesting these phenomena are indeed linked and that nonspecific binding of nitrofurantoin reactive intermediates to multiple ribosomal proteins is responsible for inhibition of overall bacterial protein synthesis.

Previous reports (13,14) indicated that an interesting phenomenon occurred at lower nitrofurantoin concentrations than those which produced inhibition of total

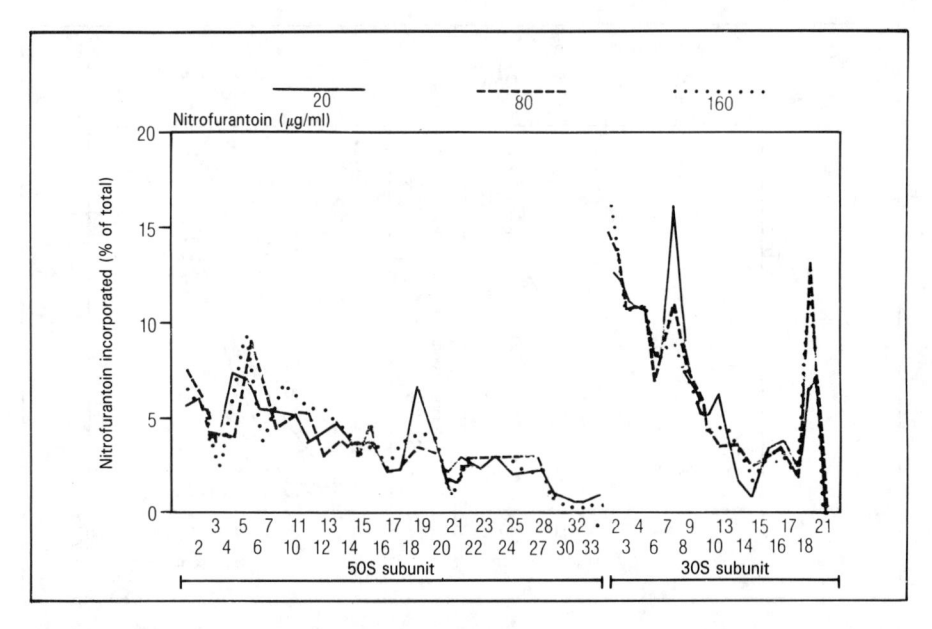

Figure 3 Escherichia coli: MRE600 were incubated with either 20, 80, or 160 µg/ml of ^{14}C-nitrofurantoin. Ribosomal proteins were then separated and radioactivity in each protein determined as described in the text.

Table 5 Ribosomal labeling by nitrofurantoin and inhibition of protein synthesis

	^{14}C-Proline incorporation (cpm)	^{14}C-Nitrofurantoin incorporation (cpm)
160 µg/ml nitrofurantoin	544	2038
160 µg/ml nitrofurantoin + 0.8% 2-mercaptoethanol	818	1192
% change due to 2-mercaptoethanol	+50.4	−41.5

Table 6 Inhibition of inducible enzyme synthesis by nitrofurantoin

	\multicolumn{3}{c}{Amount[a] of nitrofurantoin causing:}
	MIC (µg/ml)	Total growth inhibition (µg/ml)	Enzyme synthesis inhibition (µg/ml)
Escherichia coli MRE600	16	15–25	15–25[b] 14[c]
E. coli EC3669	16	15–50	15–50[b] 14[c]
E. coli 153R103	250	125–450	125–450[b]
Klebsiella pneumoniae KL-9	16	5–15	5–15[d]
Proteus vulgaris Pr-109	64	ND[c]	45[d]

[a]Highest concentration at which no inhibition was observed and lowest concentration at which inhibition was observed; [b]β-galactosidase; [c]not determined; [d]tryptophanase.

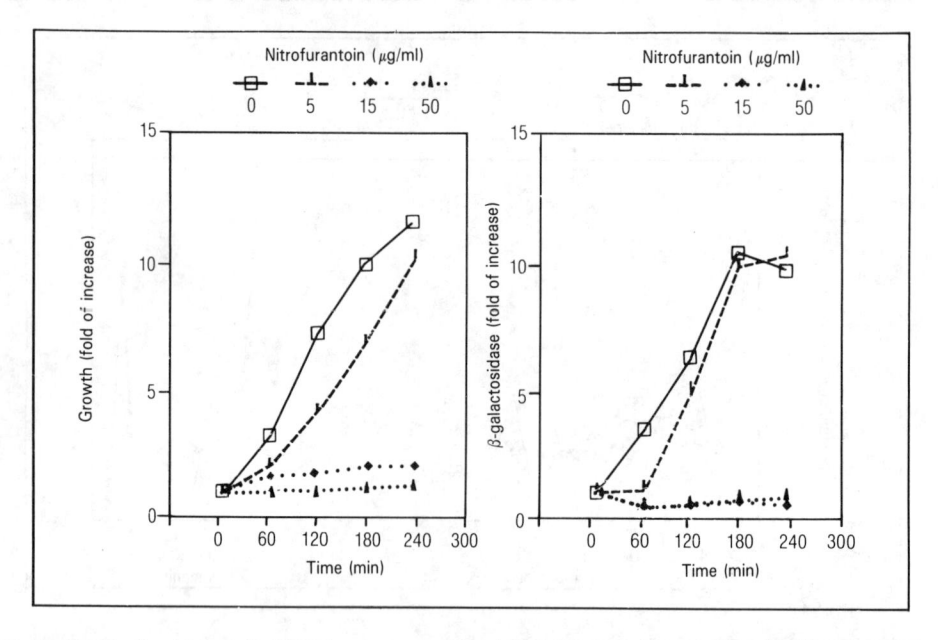

Figure 4 Escherichia coli: ES174 were grown to midlog phase, and isopropyl-β-D-thiogalactoside was added to induce β-galactosidase synthesis. After 30 min, nitrofurantoin was added as indicated, and growth and β-galactosidase activity were determined at the intervals shown.

bacterial protein synthesis. The synthesis of inducible enzymes, enzymes whose synthesis is 'turned on' by the presence of specific compounds in the bacterial growth medium, was specifically inhibited by nitrofurantoin at levels that produced no effect on total protein synthesis. This was previously demonstrated in E. coli for the enzymes β-galactosidase and galactokinase (13,14). We have now extended these observations to the synthesis of another inducible enzyme, tryptophanase, to test whether a similar effect would be seen with bacteria other than E. coli. In addition, we have shown that inhibition of inducible enzyme synthesis correlates with the MIC of nitrofurantoin for each organism and enzyme tested.

Figure 4 shows the effect of several levels of nitrofurantoin on growth and β-galactosidase synthesis in E. coli ES-174, a strain with normal susceptibility to nitrofurantoin. The levels of bacteria used here were more like those seen in clinical situations; note the low levels of nitrofurantoin that produce growth inhibition in susceptible strains under these conditions. Both effects show the same dependence on nitrofurantoin concentration. Table 6 demonstrates the correlation between growth inhibition and enzyme synthesis inhibition in other strains of E. coli (both nitrofurantoin-susceptible and resistant), as well as in K. pneumoniae and P. vulgaris.

As described earlier, incubation of ^{14}C-nitrofurantoin with E. coli resulted in the qualitatively nonspecific labeling of almost all ribosomal proteins. However, under conditions that caused inhibition of inducible enzyme synthesis, quantitative analysis of the binding data revealed that certain ribosomal proteins bound greater quantities of ^{14}C-nitrofurantoin than could be accounted for by the general increase in bound nitrofurantoin seen with increasing concentrations (Fig. 5). Interestingly, the three proteins whose labeling significantly increased under these conditions (Fig. 5, indicated by an *) reside in regions of the ribosome

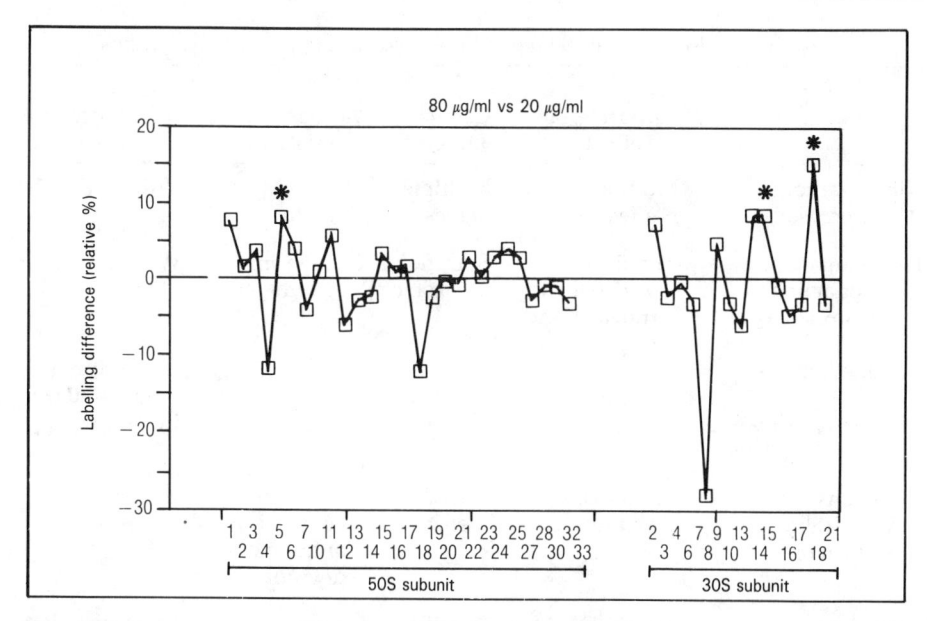

Figure 5 Escherichia coli: MRE600 were incubated with either 20 or 80 µg/ml ^{14}C-nitrofurantoin. Incorporation of radioactivity into each ribosomal protein was determined and expressed as a percentage of the total radioactivity incorporated into the respective subunit. The difference in relative labeling of a single protein at the two nitrofurantoin concentrations was then calculated and expressed as a percentage of the total absolute values of the differences observed.

believed to be involved in the initiation of messenger RNA translation into protein (15,16). Although not yet proven, this may represent another mechanism by which interaction of nitrofurantoin-reactive intermediates with ribosomal proteins can inhibit bacterial growth.

DISCUSSION

The evidence reviewed in this report indicates that the following mechanism contributes in a major way to the bactericidal effect of nitrofurantoin macrocrystals. First, nitrofurantoin is reduced within susceptible bacteria, generating highly reactive intermediates. These nitrofurantoin intermediates bind nonspecifically to almost every ribosomal protein. Given the highly ordered structure of the bacterial ribosome, it might reasonably be inferred that nitrofurantoin binding to multiple ribosomal proteins would be sufficient to disrupt ribosomal structure so as to inhibit protein synthesis. In addition, reactive intermediates of other nitrofuran antibiotics have been shown to bind to RNA associated with the ribosome, which could further disrupt its functioning (9). This leads us to propose multiple targets for the antibacterial effect of nitrofurantoin macrocrystals, only some of which may be required under a given set of conditions for antibacterial activity.

A comparison with the modes of action of other antimicrobials commonly used for treatment of uncomplicated UTIs and mechanisms by which bacteria develop resistance to them (17) indicates the potential significance of multiple target molecules (Table 7). For example, sulfonamides and trimethoprim inhibit specific enzymes involved in folic acid synthesis. A single mutagenic change can lead

Table 7 *Mechanism of action and resistance among antimicrobial agents*

	Antibacterial effect	Cellular targets	Mechanism of resistance	Degree of resistance in *Escherichia coli*
Nitrofurantoin macrocrystals	Multiple effects	Multiple sites	—	Very rare
Folate antagonists: Sulfonamides Sulfisoxazole	Inhibit folic acid pathway (nucleic acid synthesis)	Specific enzyme(s)	Change in enzyme(s)	Widespread
Trimethoprim				Limited; not widely used
Trimethoprim-sulfamethoxazole				Increasing
β-Lactams Amoxicillin Ampicillin	Inhibit cell-wall synthesis	Specific enzymes	Change in enzyme(s); antibiotic degradation	Widespread
Quinolones Norfloxacin Ciprofloxacin	Inhibit DNA synthesis	Specific enzyme	Change in permeability; change in enzyme	Unknown; not yet in long-term use

to resistance to either of these agents. Once a mutation occurs, resistance is generally persistent and irreversible (17). Sulfonamides and trimethoprim are frequently combined to reduce the development of resistance. Although resistance to the combination requires two separate events (one for each antibiotic), each event can in itself be accomplished from one mutation. In addition, strains with pre-existing resistance to either one of the components would have to undergo only a single change to become resistant to the other.

As predicted, resistance to the TMP-SMX combination is significantly lower than to either agent alone. However, a general pattern of gradually increasing resistance has been observed. Over a five-year period, resistance to TMP-SMX increased from 0.4% to 12.6% among *S. aureus* strains in one study (3). In 1982, 10% to 20% of gram-negative bacteria collected in a New York survey were resistant (4). Most disturbingly, a survey of sensitivity to TMP-SMX among strains of *E. coli* isolated in three centers in Israel detected steadily decreasing susceptibility. In 1984 and 1985, the last years of the study, only 44% to 55% of *E. coli* at these sites were sensitive, as compared with initial 75% to 79% in the same centers in 1981 (5). The β-lactam antibiotics act by inhibiting bacterial cell-wall synthesis, generally by interacting with one or two specific binding proteins. Resistance can develop (and has developed) both by alterations in these proteins and by the production of β-lactamases that degrade the drug. Although more advanced classes of these antibiotics with greater stability to β-lactamase enzymes are continually being introduced, even very stable antibiotics are functionally inactivated by these enzymes by mechanisms that are not well defined. The combination of β-lactams with β-lactamase inhibitors such as clavulanic acid can be effective against strains that produce limited quantities of β-lactamases; however, *in vivo* selection of strains elaborating greater quantities of β-lactamase enzyme would in all likelihood overcome this inhibition.

The quinolones are another class of drugs that act through a single target molecule. These agents appear to act by inhibiting DNA synthesis (8). This class of agents has great therapeutic potential, because bacteria resistant to other drug classes are generally not resistant to quinolones and vice versa. However, some clinical resistance to all of the new fluoroquinolone agents has already been encountered (7,8). Generally, strains resistant to one of the new fluoroquinolones are resistant to the entire class (7). The exact degree of resistance development associated with these agents will not be clear until they have been in broader use for several years.

Other antimicrobial classes, in addition to nitrofurans, act by inhibition of protein synthesis. Their modes of action, when known, involve binding to specific ribosomal proteins. As a consequence, single mutational events are capable of producing resistance. For example, erythromycins bind to a single protein in the 50S ribosomal subunit; resistance can arise from mutations in this component (17).

It would appear, then, that the multiple, nonspecific interactions of reactive intermediates with ribosomal proteins contribute to the singular lack of resistance development that characterizes nitrofurantoin macrocrystals. For a bacterial cell to escape the consequences of the binding of these intermediates, multiple simultaneous mutations of ribosomal proteins would be required. Because these proteins are vital to cell survival, and even minor changes in the highly ordered ribosomal structure may be lethal, this is essentially impossible. Groups capable of reaction with activated nitrofurantoin intermediates are widely distributed in proteins and other biologic macromolecules. However, it is possible to propose potential mechanisms by which resistance could occur prior to the activation of nitrofurantoin to reactive intermediates. Why are no organisms demonstrating these means of resistance encountered in clinical practice?

As one example, recall that generation of nitrofurantoin reactive intermediates requires bacterial reductase enzymes (Table 1). It is possible to derive laboratory mutant strains that show significantly diminished (Table 1) nitrofuran reductase activity (e.g., *E. coli* 153R103 in Table 1). However, this activity appears to be relatively equally distributed among several enzyme systems (9). Elimination of reductase activity would thus require several mutational events, dramatically decreasing the probability of spontaneous appearance of high-level nitrofurantoin resistance mutants, thus accounting for the nonappearance of clinically significant nitrofurantoin resistance due to loss of reductase activity.

CONCLUSION

Nitrofurantoin macrocrystals is an effective, safe, bactericidal urinary tract antibacterial and is unique among antibacterial agents for the low frequency of resistance development among pathogens within the spectrum of activity. Data obtained in this study indicate that the activity of this antibacterial results from reductive activation followed by nonspecific binding of reactive intermediates to ribosomal proteins. This in turn leads to broad-based inhibition of protein synthesis at the ribosomal level. Such a mechanism is unique to this class of antimicrobials. The large number of target proteins may explain the lack of significant resistance and at the same time suggests that the continued use of nitrofurantoin macrocrystals is extremely unlikely to result in the development of resistance in presently susceptible strains. This is in marked contrast to many of the newer, broad-spectrum agents such as the quinolones, which are already showing some resistance development. Widespread use of these agents for indications such as lower urinary tract infections may lead to the more rapid emergence of resistant strains and thereby compromise their utility for systemic and difficult-to-treat infections. In order to preserve the long-term efficacy of agents such as the quinolones, use of Macrodantin®, which is effective against more than 90% of urinary tract pathogens and does not promote resistance development, as the drug of choice for management of lower urinary tract infections seems to be strongly indicated.

REFERENCES

(1) Brumfitt W, Hamilton-Miller JMT. Bacterial resistance; how to keep it in check. *Contemp Obstet Gynecol* 1986; **27**: 149.
(2) Cobb DK. Mechanisms of resistance to extended spectrum cephalosporins. *Hosp Pract* 1986; **21**: 100T-100V.
(3) Chattopadhyay B. Co-trimoxazole resistant *Staphylococcus aureus* in hospital practice. *J Antimicrob Chemother* 1977; **3**: 371-374.
(4) Wormser GP, Keusch GT, Heel RC. Co-trimoxazole (trimethoprim-sulfamethoxazole): an updated review of its antibacterial activity and clinical efficacy. *Drugs* 1982; **24**: 459-518.
(5) Alon U, Davidai G, Berant M, Merzbach D. Five-year survey of changing patterns of susceptibility of bacterial uropathogens to trimethoprim-sulfamethoxazole and other antimicrobial agents. *Antimicrob Agents Chemother* 1987; **31**: 126-128.
(6) Fruensgaard K, Korner B. Alterations in the sensitivity pattern after use of trimethoprim-sulfamethoxazole for two years in the treatment of urinary tract infections. *Chemotherapy* 1974; **20**: 97-101.
(7) Neu HC. Bacterial resistance to fluoroquinolones. *Rev Infect Dis* 1988; **10** (suppl 1): S57-63.
(8) LeBel M. Ciprofloxacin: chemistry, mechanism of action, resistance, antimicrobial spectrum, pharmacokinetics, clinical trials, and adverse reactions. *Pharmacotherapy* 1988; **8**: 3-33.
(9) McCalla DR. Nitrofurans. In: Hahn FE, ed. *Mechanism of action of antimicrobial agents.* New York: Springer-Verlag, 1979; **9**: 176.
(10) Brumfitt W, Hamilton-Miller JMT. Development of bacterial resistance during the treatment of urinary tract infection: A constant clinical challenge. In: Schroder FH, ed. *Recent advances in the treatment of urinary tract infections.* Royal Society of Medicine Services International Congress and Symposium Series, 1985; **97**: 13-24.
(11) Yu T, McCalla DR. Effect of nitrofurazone on bacterial DNA and ribosome synthesis and on the function of ribosomes. *Chem Biol Interact* 1976; **14**: 81.
(12) Geyl D, Bock A, Isono K. An improved method of two-dimensional gel electrophoresis: Analysis of mutationally altered ribosomal proteins of *Escherichia coli*. *MGG* 1981; **181**: 309-312.
(13) Grant DJW, De Szöcs J. Inhibitory effects of some anti-inflammatory and other analgesics and nitrofurans on the induction of beta-galactosidase synthesis in *Klebsiella aerogenes*. *Biochem Pharmacol* 1971; **20**: 625-635.
(14) Herrlich P, Schweiger M. Nitrofurans, a group of synthetic antibiotics, with a new mode of action: discrimination of specific messenger RNA classes. *Proc Natl Acad Sci USA* 1976; **73**: 3386-3390.
(15) Lake JA. Evolving ribosome structure: domains in archaebacteria, eubacteria, eocytes and eukaryotes. *Ann Rev Biochem* 1985; **54**: 507-530.
(16) Capel MS, Engelman DM, Freeborn BR, et al. A complete mapping of proteins in the small ribosomal subunit of *Escherichia coli*. *Science* 1987; **238**: 1403-1406.
(17) Sande MA, Mandell GL. Antimicrobial agents. General considerations. In: Goodman AG, Goodman LS, Rall TW, Murad F, eds. *The pharmacological basis of therapeutics,* 7th ed. New York: Macmillan, 1985: 1066-1094.

A comparison of amoxicillin, co-trimoxazole, nitrofurantoin macrocrystals, and trimethoprim in the treatment of lower urinary tract infection

R. Ellis[1] and D. J. Moseley[2]

General Practitioners, [1]Leicester, and, [2]Bamford, Near Sheffield, England, UK

ABSTRACT

A randomized single-blind, parallel group study was conducted to compare the efficacy of four antibacterials used in general practice. Enrolled in the study were 390 patients, aged 18 to 40 years, with symptoms of lower urinary tract infection (LUTI). A midstream urine sample was collected before treatment, and only the results of 119 patients (31%) who had colony counts of organisms greater than 10^5/ml were evaluated for efficacy.

After seven days' treatment, amoxicillin, co-trimoxazole, nitrofurantoin macrocrystals (Macrodantin®), and trimethoprim effectively relieved the symptoms of LUTI and cleared the infecting organism in the majority of patients studied. Nitrofurantoin macrocrystals and trimethoprim were proven more effective than amoxicillin and co-trimoxazole, as fewer patients had symptoms and infecting organisms at the end of the seven-day treatment period. Treatment was successful in 94% of patients taking trimethoprim, in 93% receiving nitrofurantoin macrocrystals, in 80% receiving co-trimoxazole, and in 64% receiving amoxicillin. Some patients experienced a recurrent infection between the end of therapy on day 7 and their final follow-up visit on day 35; of these, 31% were taking co-trimoxazole, 16% trimethoprim, and 9% nitrofurantoin macrocrystals. None were receiving amoxicillin. Few patients reported adverse reactions: 13 of 390, or 3%, with no difference from one treatment to another.

Laboratory-predicted sensitivity was compared with the actual sensitivity of each isolated organism to the agent being studied. In the amoxicillin, co-trimoxazole, and trimethoprim groups, some organisms reported as resistant cleared, whereas some 'sensitive' organisms did not. However, with nitrofurantoin macrocrystals, all organisms had been eradicated by the end of the seven-day treatment period, whether they had been reported as resistant or sensitive.

INTRODUCTION

Patients whose physicians suspect a lower urinary tract infection (LUTI) are usually treated for five to 10 days. Therapy is for the symptomatic relief of dysuria and

Management of urinary tract infections, edited by Lloyd H. Harrison, 1990; Royal Society of Medicine Services International Congress and Symposium Series No. 154, published by Royal Society of Medicine Services Limited.

frequency and for eliminating the causative organisms, which have been identified by analysis of a pretreatment midstream urine (MSU) sample.

Among the antibacterials used in LUTI therapy are amoxicillin, co-trimoxazole, and trimethoprim (1-4). However, because of the widespread use of these drugs, some strains of microorganisms have developed resistance (5), thus reducing their clinical value. Therefore, as first-line therapy, an antibiotic that has produced a minimum number of strains of resistant microorganisms and, at the same time, has an appropriate spectrum of activity is desirable.

Many of the agents routinely used in the treatment of LUTI are so familiar that insufficient consideration is given to whether their efficacy has changed with time. This study was designed to assess the comparative efficacy of four such agents: amoxicillin (Amoxil®, Bencard), co-trimoxazole (Septrin®, Wellcome), nitrofurantoin macrocrystals (Macrodantin®, Norwich Eaton), and trimethoprim (Monotrim®, Duphar).

OBJECTIVES

The objectives of the study were as follows:
- To evaluate the efficacy of nitrofurantoin macrocrystals relative to amoxicillin, co-trimoxazole, and trimethoprim in the treatment of LUTI
- To identify the causative organisms responsible for the initial infections and any episodes of recurrent infection
- To determine the incidence of recurrent urinary tract infections in the four treatment groups 28 days after cessation of treatment
- To determine the incidence of side effects in the four treatment groups

PATIENTS AND METHODS

All patients enrolled in the study were women between ages 18 and 41 who had consulted their general practitioners with symptoms of dysuria and frequency suggestive of a LUTI. Among the women excluded from the study were those who had flank pain and temperatures of 38° C or higher; who had experienced more than two episodes of recurrent UTI within the preceding 12 months; who were pregnant; who had not menstruated within the previous six weeks; or who had any coexisting bronchial, hepatic, or renal disease. Also excluded were patients with a known allergy or hypersensitivity to sulfonamide, trimethoprim, co-trimoxazole, penicillin, or nitrofurantoin.

STUDY DESIGN

The trial was a single-blind, parallel group comparison to evaluate the efficacy and tolerability of amoxicillin, 250 mg t.i.d.; co-trimoxazole, two tablets, each 80 mg trimethoprim, 400 mg sulfamethoxazole, b.i.d.; nitrofurantoin macrocrystals, 100 mg q.i.d.; and trimethoprim, 200 mg b.i.d. The study was approved by the Leicester Health Authority Ethical Committee prior to commencement and conducted in accordance with the Declaration of Helsinki. Each patient gave informed consent before participating.

After baseline evaluation, patients were randomly allocated to one of the four treatment groups and given a trial pack containing their seven days of medication with full instructions for taking it and three urine specimen tubes with instructions for collecting a clean-catch MSU sample. Patients were asked to return for follow-up examinations at the end of day 7 (data are analyzed for patients returning between days 6 and 10) and again four weeks later on day 35 (data are analyzed for patients returning between days 28 and 48).

An early-morning MSU sample was taken at baseline and examined for color and turbidity by the investigator. An oxoid dipslide (MacConkey agar/cystine lactose electrolyte deficient medium) was inoculated with this sample. The urine samples and dipslides were examined by centralized laboratory facilities to provide biochemical and microscopic data, both identification and a colony count of the infecting organism, and antibiotic sensitivity and resistance data. Serotyping of isolates was not done in this study.

A colony count of organisms greater than or equal to 10^5/ml of a predominant pathogen was considered confirmation of the presence of a UTI. Patients whose colony counts were less than 10^5/ml were withdrawn from the study at day 7. For patients with confirmed LUTI, the MSU and assessment of symptoms were repeated at the end of day 7 and at follow-up on day 35. On those days the status of side effects was also recorded.

Patients were asked to complete a diary card, recording the dates and times of the first dose and when the relief of symptoms was first noted. This card was returned to the investigator at the end of treatment. The chi-squared test was used to compare the time span to relief of symptoms for each of the four treatment groups.

Treatment was considered successful when at the end of treatment the MSU sample contained infecting organisms fewer than 10^5/ml and the patient was symptom free. This was the principle measure of efficacy. The presence of symptoms and the MSU colony count after treatment and at follow-up on day 35 were summarized as frequency tables and analyzed using the chi-squared and the Fisher exact tests. Patients who were lost to follow-up were not included in the analysis of efficacy.

For each organism isolated in a pretreatment MSU sample, the central pathology laboratory routinely listed its *in vitro* sensitivity to a number of standard antimicrobial agents. These pretreatment *in vitro* sensitivities and the actual culture results of MSU samples on day 7 were listed for comparison. The nature, duration, severity, and outcome of all adverse reactions also were recorded.

RESULTS

Only 119 (31%) of the 390 patients recruited to this study had baseline colony counts of organisms greater than or equal to 10^5/ml. The remaining patients were

Table 1 Patient distribution

Agent	n	Age range (year)	Mean age (year)	SD
Amoxicillin	26	18.1–40.6	31.1	6.9
Co-trimoxazole	23	19.0–40.3	30.7	7.5
Nitrofurantoin macrocrystals	33	20.1–40.8	30.4	5.7
Trimethoprim	37	18.8–39.8	30.7	5.8

Key: n = number of patients; SD = standard deviation.

Table 2 Time span to relief of symptoms

Day from first dose	Amoxicillin	Co-trimoxazole	Nitrofurantoin macrocrystals	Trimethoprim
<1	0	1	0	3
1	2	1	3	7
2	5	6	9	8
3	4	3	5	11
4	1	2	5	3
5	3	1	3	1
6	1	1	0	0
7	0	1	0	0
Total	16	16	25	33

Table 3 Patients with symptoms

Agent	At end of treatment (day 7)	At follow-up (day 35)
Amoxicillin	5/23 (22%)	0/11 (0%)
Co-trimoxazole	2/20 (10%)	2/12 (17%)
Nitrofurantoin macrocrystals	2/28 (7%)	1/22 (5%)
Trimethoprim	1/35 (3%)	2/32 (6%)

withdrawn from the study and their data not included in the analysis for efficacy. Data from three patients were unavailable for analysis. The distribution between treatments and the mean age for each group are shown in Table 1. A few patients in each group were taking concomitant medication: ten were taking an oral contraceptive; two were receiving parenteral insulin for diabetes; four were taking benzodiazepines for sleep disorders; and one was taking a diuretic for water retention. A number of patients were lost to follow-up at day 7—one from the amoxicillin group, three from the co-trimoxazole group, five from the nitrofurantoin macrocrystals group, and two from the trimethoprim group.

Relief of symptoms

The patient diary cards of those who were treatment successes (symptom free, with colony count less than 10^5/ml) at day 7 were evaluated for time span to relief of symptoms. The distribution of results is summarized in Table 2. The difference among the treatment groups was not significant ($p=0.38$). Few patients reported symptoms at visits on days 7 or 35 (Table 3). No significant difference in the number of symptoms was reported among the treatment groups.

Colony count

Some patients failed to provide the MSU specimen at day 7, but of those who were evaluable, the proportion with colony counts of organisms greater than or equal to 10^5/ml in the co-trimoxazole and amoxicillin groups was higher than that in either the trimethoprim or nitrofurantoin macrocrystals groups (Table 4). These differences were of statistical significance between nitrofurantoin macrocrystals and both co-trimoxazole ($p=0.05$) and amoxicillin ($p=0.013$) and between trimethoprim and amoxicillin ($p=0.03$).

Table 4 *Patients with colony counts greater than 10^5/ml*

Agent	At end of treatment (day 7)	At follow-up (day 35)
Amoxicillin	6/24 (25%)	0/11 (0%)
Co-trimoxazole	4/20 (20%)	2/13 (15%)
Nitrofurantoin macrocrystals	0/28 (0%)	1/22 (5%)
Trimethoprim	1/35 (3%)	3/32 (9%)

Table 5 *Results of treatment*

Agent	Success	95% Confidence limits for proportions of successes
Amoxicillin	16/25 (64%)	45% to 83%
Co-trimoxazole	16/20 (80%)	62% to 98%
Nitrofurantoin macrocrystals	26/28 (93%)	83% to 100%
Trimethoprim	33/35 (94%)	86% to 100%

Success of treatment

Only patients who at day 7 were symptom free and had a colony count less than 10^5/ml were considered treatment successes. The proportion of patients who were treated successfully in each group were: amoxicillin 64%, co-trimoxazole 80%, nitrofurantoin macrocrystals 93%, and trimethoprim 94% (Table 5). Statistically, success of treatment was significantly higher for nitrofurantoin macrocrystals ($p=0.023$) and trimethoprim ($p=0.008$) compared with amoxicillin.

Recurrence of infection

Patients were considered to be reinfected or to have had a recurrent infection if, after successful treatment, their symptoms returned or they had a colony count of a predominant organism in their urine of greater than or equal to 10^5/ml. As organisms identified in the MSU samples were not serotyped, distinction could not be drawn between episodes of reinfection and relapse. Recurrent symptoms or colony counts of greater than or equal to 10^5/ml occurred in none of the 11 patients who had taken amoxicillin, in four of 13 (31%) who had taken co-trimoxazole, two of 22 (9%) who had received nitrofurantoin macrocrystals, and five of 32 (16%) who had taken trimethoprim (Table 6). There were no statistically significant differences among these reinfection rates ($p>0.1$, the Fisher exact test).

Table 6 *Incidence of recurrent infection*

Agent	Incidence of recurrent infection[a]	95% Confidence limits for proportions of recurrent infection
Amoxicillin	0/11 (0%)	—
Co-trimoxazole	4/13 (31%)	5% to 57%
Nitrofurantoin macrocrystals	2/22 (9%)	0% to 22%
Trimethoprim	5/32 (16%)	3% to 29%

[a] *Differences in incidence are not statistically significant. Incidence is based upon patients' data collected between study days 28 and 48.*

Table 7 *Organisms isolated from urine cultures*

Organism	Day 0 (n=119)	Day 7 (n=107)	Day 35 (n=78)
Escherichia coli	82	8	5
Coliforms	20	1	—
Streptococcus sp	12	—	—
Klebsiella sp	2	2	—
Staphylococcus sp	1	—	1
Proteus sp	2	—	—

Table 8 In vitro *sensitivities vs actual results*

		Culture results—day 7	
In vitro sensitivity (day 0)	Total patients	Organisms still present	Organisms eradicated
Amoxicillin			
Resistant	8	2	6
Sensitive	14	2	12
Co-trimoxazole			
Resistant	3	0	3
Sensitive	15	2	13
Nitrofurantoin macrocrystals			
Resistant	6	0	6
Sensitive	22	0	22
Trimethoprim			
Resistant	5	1	4
Sensitive	29	0	29

Infecting organisms

Table 7 summarizes the organisms isolated from MSU samples at baseline day (day 1), day 7, and day 35. Of the 119 positive baseline MSU samples, 82 (69%) contained *Escherichia coli*. Coliforms and *Streptococcus* sp were the next most frequently isolated organisms, 17% and 10%, respectively. At the end of treatment at day 7, most patients' urine showed no growth (18 amoxicillin, 16 co-trimoxazole, 28 nitrofurantoin macrocrystals, 34 trimethoprim). Of those patients still infected at day 7, *E. coli* was the principal causative organism, accounting for eight of the 11 persisting infections. The same pattern of results was seen in the day 35 samples with five of the six colony counts greater than or equal to 10^5/ml caused by *E. coli*.

For each organism isolated, the pathology laboratory routinely listed *in vitro* sensitivity to a number of standard agents. Table 8 shows a comparison of the predicted sensitivities of organisms isolated at baseline with actual sensitivities as assessed by the presence/absence of the initial infecting organism in the day 7 MSU sample. Discrepancies were noted in all four treatment groups. In all groups, the majority of organisms reported as resistant at baseline were eradicated by treatment (19 of 22). In the amoxicillin and co-trimoxazole groups, a small proportion of organisms reported as sensitive at baseline were not eradicated by treatment. In the nitrofurantoin macrocrystals group, all infecting organisms were eradicated by treatment regardless of the reported *in vitro* sensitivity at baseline.

Table 9 *Adverse reactions*

Treatment group	Adverse event	Severity	Outcome
Amoxicillin	Vaginitis	—	—
Co-trimoxazole	Nausea	Mild	Recovered
	General irritant macular rash	Severe	Still under treatment
	Skin sensitivity	Severe	Recovered
Nitrofurantoin macrocrystals	Nausea	—	—
	Vomiting	Severe	Recovered
	Hepatitis	Moderate	Recovered
	Nausea	Mild	Recovered
Trimethoprim	Nausea/vomiting	Moderate	Recovered
	Rash	Mild	Recovered
	Headaches	Mild/moderate	Recovered
	Nausea	—	—

Adverse reactions

Data from all 390 patients who entered the study were evaluated. Thirteen adverse reactions were reported (Table 9), which were evenly distributed among the groups. In the group taking amoxicillin, two patients developed vaginitis. Among those who were administered co-trimoxazole, there was one instance each of nausea, general macular rash, and skin sensitivity. In the group taking nitrofurantoin macrocrystals, two patients had nausea, a third experienced some vomiting, and another developed non-A, non-B hepatitis, which resolved three weeks after its onset. Hepatitis is a known, although rare, adverse reaction to nitrofurantoin. The presence of a three-week time delay between end of treatment and onset of the hepatic event suggests that this patient's hepatitis was unlikely to be drug related; however, a causal relationship cannot be excluded with absolute certainty. Four women in the trimethoprim group had adverse reactions. Two experienced nausea and vomiting, one developed a rash, and one had a headache.

DISCUSSION

An oral compound for use in treating LUTI ideally should attain an adequate bactericidal drug concentration in the urinary tract without affecting the ecologic balance of normal flora in other parts of the body. If swift, complete absorption and excretion do not occur, residual drug reaching the lower gut can alter the normal bowel flora, resulting in an overgrowth of *Candida* or other organisms. In short, it is desirable to use a drug whose distribution and excretion profile allow it to concentrate primarily in the urinary tract.

Nitrofurantoin macrocrystals most closely approximates the desirable features of an ideal drug of first choice for treating LUTI. Nitrofurantoin macrocrystals is rapidly and completely absorbed. The agent has a low, nonbactericidal serum concentration and a short serum half-life of only 19 min and achieves high urinary concentrations (6).

The urinary tract specificity of this agent may be the reason why the compound has shown minimal alteration of resistance profile since it first became available about 30 years ago. Nitrofurantoin macrocrystals continues to be highly effective therapy that clinicians can prescribe with confidence for both initial and recurrent UTIs.

CONCLUSIONS

This study suggests that nitrofurantoin macrocrystals and trimethoprim are more clinically effective than amoxicillin or co-trimoxazole for the treatment of LUTI.

The ideal antibiotic for treatment of uncomplicated LUTI is completely absorbed from the upper gastrointestinal tract, achieves high urinary and low systemic levels, does not alter the normal bowel or vaginal flora, and possesses a low order of toxicity. Nitrofurantoin macrocrystals has all of these qualities. Although the drug has been used for more than 30 years, the number of bacterial strains that have acquired resistance remains very small. Its clinical efficacy is high against most common uropathogens. Nitrofurantoin macrocrystals may therefore be considered a most suitable first line therapy for LUTI.

ACKNOWLEDGMENTS

We thank Norwich Eaton Ltd for their help in this project and Dr David Hutchinson (Brookwood Medical Ltd) and Mrs Carol Lewis (Norwich Eaton) for help in preparing this paper.

REFERENCES

(1) Andrewes DA, Chuter PJ, Dawson MJ, et al. Trimethoprim and co-trimoxazole in the treatment of acute urinary tract infections: patient compliance and efficacy. *J R Coll Gen Pract* 1981; **31**: 274–278.
(2) Belsheim J, Gnarpe H, Helleberg A, Svensson A. Clinical study of co-trimazine in urinary tract infections: a comparison with nitrofurantoin. *Infection* 1979; **7**: S411–413.
(3) Grob PR, Beynon GP, Gibbs FJ, Manners BT. Comparative trial of amoxicillin and cotrimoxazole in the treatment of urinary-tract infection. *Practitioner* 1977; **219**: 258–263.
(4) Ronald AR, Jagdis FA, Harding GKM, et al. Amoxicillin therapy of acute urinary infections in adults. *Antimicrob Agents Chemother* 1977; **11**: 780–784.
(5) Brumfitt W, Hamilton-Miller JMT. Development of bacterial resistance during treatment of urinary tract infections: a constant clinical challenge. In: Schröder FH, ed. *Recent advances in the treatment of urinary tract infections*. London: Royal Society of Medicine Services Limited. International Congress and Symposium Series No. 97; 1985: 13–24.
(6) Corriere JN Jr. Drug therapy and urinary tract infections: biodistribution and clinical activity of nitrofurantoin macrocrystals. In: Schröder FH, ed. *Recent advances in the treatment of urinary tract infections*. London: Royal Society of Medicine Services Limited. International Congress and Symposium Series No. 97; 1985: 7–12.

Prospective randomized comparison of the therapeutic efficacy and safety of nitrofurantoin macrocrystals vs norfloxacin in the treatment of acute symptomatic uncomplicated UTIs in women: A prelimary report

G. Harding, L. Nicolle, C. Hawkins, P. Mirwaldt and A. Ronald

Departments of Medicine & Medical Microbiology and Family Practice,
University of Manitoba, Winnipeg, Manitoba, Canada

ABSTRACT

In an ongoing study, women with acute, symptomatic, uncomplicated, lower urinary tract infections were randomized to receive nitrofurantoin macrocrystals (Macrodantin®), 50 mg po, q.i.d., or norfloxacin 400 mg po, b.i.d., for seven days of therapy. To date 50 women of a total expected study population of 100 have been recruited. Forty-two patients were evaluable for efficacy. Seven of the eight unevaluable patients had a pretherapy count of colony forming units (CFU) $<10^8/l$ of urine. The infecting organisms isolated from the evaluable patients in the nitrofurantoin macrocrystals and norfloxacin treatment groups, respectively, were: *Escherichia coli* 19, 15; *Klebsiella pneumoniae* 0, 2; *K. oxytoca* 0, 1; *Citrobacter diversus* 0, 1; *Enterobacter cloacae* 1, 0; *Staphylococcus haemolyticus* 1, 0; and *S. epidermidis* 1, 2. Two infecting organisms were isolated from one of the 42 patients. For the 42 evaluable patients the cure rates determined at five to 10 days posttherapy were 20 of 22 (91%) for patients receiving nitrofurantoin macrocrystals and 19 of 20 (95%) for patients receiving norfloxacin. Three reinfections occurred in each of the treatment groups. Two of 22 patients relapsed following nitrofurantoin macrocrystals therapy and one following norfloxacin therapy. Of the 50 patients enrolled in the study to date, two receiving nitrofurantoin macrocrystals developed nausea; of those receiving norfloxacin therapy, one developed vaginal itching and another yeast vaginitis. No adverse effect necessitated discontinuation of the study medication. There were no significant differences in outcome or adverse experiences between the two treatment groups. In this study population, nitrofurantoin macrocrystals was as effective and well-tolerated as norfloxacin for therapy of acute, symptomatic, uncomplicated, lower urinary tract infections in women.

Management of urinary tract infections, edited by Lloyd H. Harrison, 1990; Royal Society of Medicine Services International Congress and Symposium Series No. 154, published by Royal Society of Medicine Services Limited.

INTRODUCTION

More than 5 million physician-visits per year in the United States are attributable to acute symptomatic uncomplicated urinary tract infections (UTIs) (1). Nitrofurantoin macrocrystals (Macrodantin®) is a well-established, effective antimicrobial agent against the gram-negative or gram-positive organisms that are usually isolated from patients with UTIs (2). Resistance to nitrofurantoin during therapy rarely develops (3). Norfloxacin is the first of the 4-quinolone antimicrobial agents to be generally available in North America. Taken orally, it is rapidly absorbed, and urinary recovery is 30% of an oral dose of 400 mg after 48 h with peak urinary concentrations in excess of 400 mg/l (4). Norfloxacin's wide spectrum of *in vitro* activity includes gram-negative and gram-positive urinary pathogens (5). Norfloxacin has recently been shown to be effective therapy for acute UTIs (6,7).

This study is a prospective, controlled, randomized, single-blind comparison of the efficacy, tolerance, and safety of orally administered nitrofurantoin macrocrystals and norfloxacin in the therapy of acute, symptomatic, uncomplicated lower UTIs in 100 outpatients.

PATIENT SELECTION

Candidates for entry into the study were ambulatory female outpatients whose symptoms and signs suggested an acute lower UTI.

The following factors excluded patients from the study:
- Allergy to nalidixic acid or its derivatives, or to nitrofurantoin
- Pregnancy
- Sexual activity using no effective means of birth control
- Known renal impairment
- Structural abnormalities of the urinary tract
- Receipt of anti-infective medication within the five days prior to evaluation for study enrollment
- Evidence of an upper UTI.

Once written informed consent was obtained, patients were randomized to receive nitrofurantoin macrocrystals, 50 mg po, qid, or norfloxacin, 400 mg po, bid, for seven days.

PATIENT ASSESSMENT

Patients were assessed clinically before therapy, during therapy at two to four days, and posttherapy at two to three days and five to 10 days. A clean-catch, midstream urine (MSU) sample for bacteriologic culture and antimicrobial susceptibility testing was obtained before therapy and at each follow-up visit. Patients were given a diary to fill out daily, indicating the presence of symptoms, when study medication was taken, and tolerance to the antimicrobial agent. At follow-up, patients were interviewed for clinical adverse side effects.

To be evaluable for drug effectiveness, women had to have a clean-catch MSU culture containing $\geq 10^8$ CFU/l of a urinary pathogen that was not resistant to either study medication. All patients enrolled were evaluated for adverse drug effects.

BACTERIOLOGY

Standard microbiologic procedures were used to identify all isolates and a standardized test was done for agar disc diffusion susceptibility (8). Susceptibility discs contained either nitrofurantoin macrocrystals, 300 µg, or norfloxacin, 10 µg. The zone diameter of ≤14 mm indicated resistance to nitrofurantoin, and a ≤12 mm diameter indicated resistance to norfloxacin. To determine the absolute white cell count of the urine specimens, the hemocytometer counting chamber method was used.

DEFINITIONS OF OUTCOME

A cure was defined as amelioration of symptoms and signs and negative follow-up urine cultures for the pretherapy infecting organism during therapy and at two to three days and five to 10 days posttherapy. A reinfection was characterized as a negative urine culture during therapy with a urine culture $\geq 10^8$ CFU/l for a *different* organism posttherapy. A relapse comprised a negative urine culture during therapy and a positive urine culture $\geq 10^8$ CFU/l posttherapy for the same pretherapy infecting organism. The continued presence of the pretherapy infecting organism during treatment was deemed failure. Proportions were analyzed statistically with the Fisher exact test. Comparison of means was by the student *t*-test.

RESULTS

Fifty women have been entered into the study. Eight were unevaluable; 42 were evaluated for drug effectiveness. The characteristics of the patient population are compared in Table 1. There were no significant differences in any parameter.

The infecting organisms isolated from the two treatment groups are listed in Table 2. One person had two infecting organisms. *Escherichia coli* was the

Table 1 *Comparison of characteristics of population*

	Nitrofurantoin macrocrystals	Norfloxacin
Patients entered (No.)	23	27
Patients unevaluable (No.)	1	7
Reason unevaluable		
No growth	1	1
<10^8 CFUs/l	0	5
Protocol violation	0	1[a]
Patients evaluable (No.)	22	20
AgeT		
Mean ± SD	39 ± 17.0	33.9 ± 15.9
Range	20–77	18–66
Median	33.5	26.5
Females/males	22/0	20/0
No. with pyuria (cells ≥ 8×10^6/l)/No. tested	18/20	17/19

[a]Noted to have renal calculi
Key: CFUs = colony-forming units; SD = standard deviation.

Table 2 *Infecting organisms*

	Isolates (No.)	
	Nitrofurantoin macrocrystals	Norfloxacin
Gram-negative bacilli		
Escherichia coli	19	15
Klebsiella pneumoniae	0	2
K. oxytoca[a]	0	1
Citrobacter diversus	0	1
Enterobacter cloacae	1	0
Gram-positive cocci		
Staphylococcus haemolyticus	1	0
S. epidermidis	1	2
Antibody-coated bacteria		
Positive	4	4
Negative	16	13
Unavailable	2	1
Nonspecific fluorescence	0	2

[a]Mixed infection with E. coli.

Table 3 *Outcome of therapy*

	Nitrofurantoin macrocrystals	Norfloxacin
Evaluable (No.)	22	20
Cured (No./%)	20 (91%)	19 (95%)[a]
Reinfections	3	3
Relapses (No.)	2	1

[a]p Value = 0.87 by the Fisher exact test.

Table 4 *Comparison of clinical adverse drug effects[a]*

	Nitrofurantoin macrocrystals (n=23)[b]	Norfloxacin (n=27)[b]
Nausea	2	0
Vaginal itching	0	1
Yeast vaginitis	0	1

[a]No adverse effect necessitated discontinuation of study medication; [b]Number enrolled in the study.

predominant infecting organism in both groups. No major differences were seen in the type of infecting organisms or in the proportion of patients who had positive antibody-coated-bacteria tests in either treatment category.

Table 3 summarizes the outcome of therapy. As noted earlier, no significant differences were noted in the outcome of therapy between the two treatment groups. Twenty of 22 (91%) patients were cured of their pretherapy infecting organisms with nitrofurantoin macrocrystals compared with 19 of 20 (95%) with norfloxacin. Three patients experienced reinfections in each treatment group.

Table 4 lists the clinical adverse effects that were noted among the 50 persons enrolled. Two patients in each treatment group experienced adverse clinical effects, none of which necessitated the discontinuation of the study medication.

DISCUSSION

Nitrofurantoin macrocrystals is a well-established effective antimicrobial agent for UTI therapy (2). Norfloxacin, the first of the newer 4-quinolones to be generally available in North America, has also been recently shown effective for UTI therapy (6,7). This study was designed as a prospective, controlled, randomized, single-blind comparison of the efficacy, tolerance, and safety of orally administered nitrofurantoin macrocrystals and norfloxacin in the therapy of acute, symptomatic, uncomplicated, lower UTIs in outpatient women. There was no difference in outcome with the two study medications. The type 2 error would be large because of the small number of patients enrolled to date. Both nitrofurantoin macrocrystals and norfloxacin were well-tolerated. Ludwig and Pauthner were also unable to show a significant difference in the bacterial eradication rates between ofloxacin and nitrofurantoin therapy in patients with lower UTIs (9).

Because nitrofurantoin macrocrystals was as effective and well-tolerated as norfloxacin and the cost of its regimen is approximately one third that of the norfloxacin regimen, nitrofurantoin macrocrystals should remain a first-line therapy of acute, symptomatic, uncomplicated UTIs in women.

REFERENCES

(1) National Center for Health Statistics. Ambulatory medical care rendered in physicians' offices: United States, 1975. *Adv Data* 1977; **12**: 1–12.
(2) Kalowski S, Radford N, Kincaid-Smith P. Crystalline and macrocrystalline nitrofurantoin in the treatment of urinary tract infection. *N Engl J Med* 1973; **290**: 385–387.
(3) Turck M, Ronald AR, Petersdorf RG. Susceptibility of Enterobacteriaceae to nitrofurantoin correlated with eradication of bacteriuria. *Antimicrob Agents Chemother* 1966; **6**: 446–452.
(4) Sabbaj J, Hoagland VL, Shim WJ. Multiclinic comparative study of norfloxacin and TMP/SMX for treatment of urinary tract infections. *Antimicrob Agents Chemother* 1985; **27**: 297–301.
(5) Haase DA, Harding GK, Thomson MJ, Kennedy JK, Urias BA, Ronald AR. Comparative trial of norfloxacin and TMP/SMX in the treatment of women with localized, acute symptomatic urinary tract infections and antimicrobial effect on periurethral and fecal microflora. *Antimicrob Agents Chemother* 1984; **26**: 481–484.
(6) Swanson BN, Boppana VK, Vlasses PH, Rotemsch HH, Ferguson RK. Norfloxacin disposition after sequentially increasing oral doses. *Antimicrob Agents Chemother* 1983; **23**: 284–288.
(7) Haase D, Urias B, Harding G, Ronald A. Comparative *in vitro* activity of norfloxacin against urinary tract pathogens. *Eur J Clin Microbiol* 1983; **2**: 235–241.
(8) National Committee for Clinical Laboratory Standards. *Performance standards for antimicrobial disk susceptibility tests*. 3rd edn. Approved Standard M2-A3. 1983; 4(16): 373–378.
(9) Ludwig G, Pauthner H. Clinical experience with ofloxacin in upper and lower urinary tract infections: a comparison with cotrimoxazole and nitrofurantoin. *Drugs* 1987; **34** (Suppl 1): 95–99.

Preventive therapy in urinary tract infection: Twenty years' experience

W. Brumfitt[1,2] and J. M. T. Hamilton-Miller[2]

[1]Urinary Infection Clinic, [2]Department of Medical Microbiology, The Royal Free Hospital School of Medicine, University of London, London, UK

ABSTRACT

Administration of low-dose, long-term therapy to women suffering from recurrent urinary tract infection may produce a fivefold or greater decrease in the frequency of infections and a considerable improvement in their quality of life. Rational criteria suggest antibiotics for low-dose, long-term therapy should be active against the most common urinary pathogens, cause only infrequent and mild side-effects, not select for bacterial resistance, and be of low cost. Antibiotics frequently used for low-dose, long-term therapy include nitrofurantoin macrocrystals (Macrodantin®), methenamine salts, trimethoprim, and trimethoprim-sulfamethoxazole (TMP-SMX). The results of long-term comparative trials in the United Kingdom indicate nitrofurantoin macrocrystals is more effective than methenamine salts or trimethoprim in preventing recurrent infection. Long-term use of trimethoprim causes resistance in the gut flora and breakthrough infections by these resistant organisms. Studies in the United States, however, showed nitrofurantoin macrocrystals and trimethoprim-sulfamethoxazole were equally effective. This difference is explained by the more common occurrence of trimethoprim resistance in the United Kingdom than in the United States. Recent additional data suggest that nitrofurantoin macrocrystals and norfloxacin are of equivalent efficacy in low-dose, long-term therapy of recurrent urinary tract infection.

INTRODUCTION

Treatment of uncomplicated urinary tract infection (UTI) generally results in high rates of both symptomatic (clinical) cure and microbiologic eradication. Urinary infection in female patients has been claimed to be associated with a recurrence rate of approximately 20%, and some 3% to 5% of patients will suffer from multiple recurrent infections (1,2). However, little published data exists; and a recurrence rate of 20% seems to be unduly high. Low-dose, long-term therapy with an appropriate antimicrobial has been convincingly demonstrated to be successful in preventing recurrence in many of these patients (3,4). Low-dose, long-term therapy may be begun after the urine is sterilized and is most often continued for three to 12 months. Several antibiotics have been found effective for this purpose, including nitrofurantoin macrocrystals (3,5–7), trimethoprim (4), and the urinary antiseptic methenamine (5,8). The combination of trimethoprim and sulfamethoxazole has also been used with success (4,9). Recently, norfloxacin has been considered for low-dose, long-term therapy (10). A series of clinical trials have been performed to compare the safety and efficacy of these antibiotics, as well as to develop rational dosage schedules and guidelines for their use. The results of these trials are reviewed below.

THE PROBLEM OF RECURRENCE

The rate of recurrence after the first episode of uncomplicated UTI has been estimated to be as high as 20% (1,11) although in the authors' experience it is usually about 10%. For obvious reasons such epidemiologic data is difficult to obtain.

The term recurrence actually refers to two different types of events (12). The first, relapse, may be defined as a second isolation of the original infecting strain, and may result from failure of the antibiotic to eradicate the pathogen completely. This, in turn, can be caused by an inadequate course of therapy, poor compliance, involvement of the upper urinary tract, or the presence of urologic abnormalities or underlying disease.

Possible abnormalities whose presence may predispose to relapse include renal calculi, obstruction, vesicoureteric reflux and, in man, chronic bacterial prostatitis. Failure to eradicate the infecting organism may be evident during treatment (persistence) or up to six weeks posttreatment when the organism may reappear.

The second type of recurrence is reinfection, defined as the isolation of a new pathogenic strain. According to reports, reinfection is much more common than relapse among young, healthy women (13); our own data do not support this. However, without detailed strain identification, including serotyping, this distinction between reinfection and relapse cannot be made (14). Although some reinfections undoubtedly arise following colonization of the vagina and perineum with gram-negative bacilli, this is by no means always the case (15). Antibiotics that select for resistance in *Escherichia coli* in the intestine may lead to such colonization by resistant strains (3,16,17).

INDICATIONS AND ANTIBIOTIC SELECTION

The terms preventive therapy, secondary prevention (4), and low-dose, long-term therapy (18) have all been used interchangeably to describe chronic administration of antibiotics to prevent the recurrence of urinary tract infections following eradication of the original infection. Low-dose, long-term therapy is clearly beneficial for preventing recurrences in prepubertal girls (19,20), pregnant women (21), and elderly men (22). However, most studies have been in nonpregnant female patients (who commonly suffer recurrent UTIs). The principal advantage of preventive treatment for these patients is improved quality of life, including relief of symptoms; improved job attendance; and an increase in sexual harmony (23). Low-dose, long-term therapy using appropriate antibiotics and dosage schedules is a highly cost-effective and more humane alternative to withholding antibiotics until there is a symptomatic complaint.

Only a few of the many antibiotics frequently employed in acute urinary infection also meet the criteria for low-dose, long-term therapy. The agent must be active against the common urinary pathogens and have a low incidence of side-effects to be acceptable for chronic administration. Second, it must not allow resistant strains to appear in the bowel flora. Third, it should be inexpensive. An antibiotic with these attributes will be effective and should be acceptable to patients, thus assuring good compliance.

According to these criteria, sulfonamides, tetracyclines, and amoxicillin are contraindicated because they frequently result in the development of resistant strains in the feces during long-term administration. Consequently, breakthrough infections are likely even when the bladder urine contains 'adequate' concentrations of antibiotics (24). The role of oral cephalosporins in low-dose, long-term therapy needs further study; doses of cephalexin and cephradine, 250 mg daily, have been reported to be effective (25,26).

The agents that best meet the criteria for low-dose, long-term therapy are nitrofurantoin macrocrystals, trimethoprim, TMP-SMX, and methenamine mandelate or hippurate. The new fluoroquinolone, norfloxacin, 100 mg at night, has also been suggested as a suitable low-dose, long-term therapy (10).

DOSAGE

Adequate low-dose, long-term therapy does not require the urine to continuously contain effective antibacterial levels. Rather, a single dose at bedtime seems highly effective and may be optimal, as it allows maximum antibiotic concentrations to remain in the bladder overnight. However, for agents with relatively long half-lives such as trimethoprim and norfloxacin, continuous levels are probably obtained with a single daily dose. Most clinical experience is with one fourth of the usual therapeutic dose (3), although lower doses (for example, one eighth of the therapeutic dose) (7) have also been used.

COMPARATIVE CLINICAL TRIALS OF ANTIBIOTIC LOW-DOSE, LONG-TERM THERAPY

Four representative clinical trials of low-dose, long-term therapy will be reviewed. In the first, nitrofurantoin (not in the macrocrystalline formulation) was compared with methenamine hippurate (5). Ninety-five female patients with recurrent UTI were treated with either methenamine hippurate, 1 g every 12 h, or nitrofurantoin, 50 mg every 12 h for up to one year. In this and subsequent studies, the groups were statistically similar in age, number, and frequency of previous symptomatic attacks, and presence of underlying structural abnormalities as detected by radiologic examination. Since the length of time of low-dose, long-term antibiotic administration differed considerably among patients, comparison of efficacy was made by determining both the absolute number of attacks and the intervals between symptomatic or documented infections.

Measured against the frequency of breakthrough bacteriuria, nitrofurantoin was more than twice as effective as methenamine (Table 1) and reduced the frequency of attacks 6.4-fold compared with the pretreatment attack rate. Five microbiologically documented infections were found in patients treated with nitrofurantoin, and 25 among those treated with methenamine hippurate. Similarly, nitrofurantoin was more effective in lessening the occurrence of

Table 1 *Comparative efficacy of low-dose, long-term therapy with nitrofurantoin and methenamine hippurate[a]*

	Nitrofurantoin	Methenamine hippurate
Number of evaluable patients	43	56
Total patient days of therapy	9680	16 032
Number of bacteriuric episodes while on treatment	5	25
Percent of patients with no bacteriuric episodes	91%	67%
Mean interval between bacteriuric episodes (days)	1936	640
Number of symptomatic episodes while on treatment	27	102
Percent of patients with no symptomatic episodes	58%	27%
Mean interval between symptomatic episodes (days)	358.5	157

[a]*Dosage schedule: nitrofurantoin, 50 mg, or methenamine hippurate, 1 g, every 12 h. (Data from reference 5.)*

symptoms of infection—dysuria and frequency of urination. All five breakthrough infections during nitrofurantoin therapy were caused by *E. coli* (the strains involved were sensitive to nitrofurantoin), as were 21 of 25 infections in patients treated with methenamine. The other breakthrough infections in the methenamine-treated group were caused by enterococci (two strains), *Staphylococcus epidermidis*, micrococci, and *Serratia* sp. Interestingly, the incidence of symptomatic recurrence among 29 patients after they had stopped low-dose, long-term treatment was similar to that during the trial and was much less than the pretrial incidence. This indicates that low-dose, long-term therapy for one year made patients less liable to recurrence after stopping low-dose, long-term therapy. Side effects and drug discontinuation due to side effects (usually nausea) were significantly more common in nitrofurantoin-treated patients. The rate of side effects observed with nitrofurantoin was 40%, which was significantly greater than that observed in a later trial (3) using the macrocrystalline form of the drug. However, different dosage schedules were used in the two studies (3,5).

Table 2 *Comparative efficacy of low-dose, long-term therapy with nitrofurantoin macrocrystals and trimethoprim[a]*

	Nitrofurantoin macrocrystals	Trimethoprim
Number of evaluable patients	34	38
Total patient days of therapy	10 965	10 149
Number of bacteriuric episodes while on treatment	5	28
Percent of patients with no bacteriuric episodes	88%	58%
Mean interval between bacteriuric episodes (days)	2193	362
Number of symptomatic episodes while on treatment	37	47
Percent of patients with no symptomatic episodes	62%	34%
Mean interval between symptomatic episodes (days)	296.4	215.9

[a]*Dosage schedule: nitrofurantoin macrocrystals, 100 mg, or trimethoprim, 100 mg, nightly. (Data from reference 3.)*

Table 3 *Efficacy of nitrofurantoin macrocrystals as low-dose, long-term therapy in patients with and without radiologic abnormalities*[a]

	No abnormality	Abnormality
Number of evaluable patients	26	8
Percent of patients with no bacteriuric episodes	88.5%	88%
Percent of patients with no symptomatic episodes	61.5%	63%

[a]*Dosage schedule: nitrofurantoin macrocrystals, 100 mg, nightly. (Data from reference 3.)*

In the second trial, we compared nitrofurantoin macrocrystals with trimethoprim (3). Trimethoprim alone was preferred to TMP-SMX because the incidence of sulfonamide resistance was high and a significant proportion of patients were allergic to sulfonamide (27). Each drug was given at night, 100 mg, to patients with a history of frequently recurring infections. Urine culture confirmed that all patients had been cured of their most recent infection. Many had suffered six to 12 infections in the preceding year. No significant demographic difference between the groups was detected. As shown in Table 2, nitrofurantoin macrocrystals were considerably more effective than trimethoprim in preventing bacteriuria and symptomatic attacks. Notably, the effectiveness of low-dose, long-term therapy was not reduced in patients with underlying radiologic abnormalities found on intravenous urography (Table 3). Side effects, usually nausea, were greater with macrocrystalline nitrofurantoin, and more patients stopped taking the drug. However, most of the discontinuations in the nitrofurantoin group occurred within a few days of enrollment. Thus, the drug is ultimately tolerated by the most patients who did not experience adverse effects soon after initiation of treatment. Note that four trimethoprim-treated patients withdrew because of

Table 4 *Species and resistance patterns of organisms causing breakthrough infections during low-dose, long-term therapy with nitrofurantoin macrocrystals or trimethoprim*[a]

Therapy	No.[b] of patients	Infective organisms (No.)	Resistance to trimethoprim	Resistance to sulfonamides	Resistance to nitrofurantoin
Trimethoprim	28	Escherichia coli (21) Staphylococcus epidermidis (5) Streptococcus faecalis (1) Enterobacter cloacae (1)	82%	61%	0
Nitrofurantoin macrocrystals	5	E. coli (4) Klebsiella pneumoniae (1)	20%	40%	0

[a]*Dosage schedule: nitrofurantoin macrocrystals, 100 mg, or trimethoprim, 100 mg, nightly;* [b]*Number of breakthrough infections. (Data from reference 3.)*

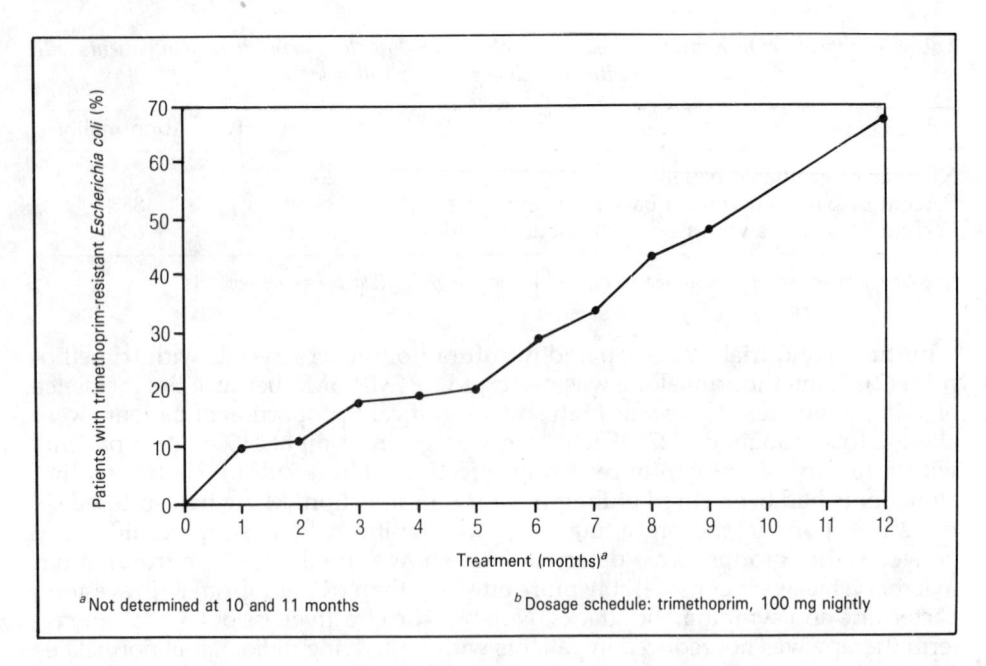

Figure 1 *The graph shows an increase of the number of patients with trimethoprim-resistant* Escherichia coli *detected in the periurethral region during low-dose, long-term therapy with trimethoprim[b]. (Data from reference 3.)*

[a] Not determined at 10 and 11 months   [b] Dosage schedule: trimethoprim, 100 mg nightly

multiple breakthrough infections with resistant pathogens, which did not occur with nitrofurantoin macrocrystals.

The organisms that cause breakthrough infections and their resistance patterns are described in Table 4. Most recurrences were due to *E. coli*. Particularly significant is that most breakthrough infections in the trimethoprim group were caused by trimethoprim-resistant organisms, because trimethoprim selected for resistant strains of *E. coli* in the feces. Such strains were acquired by an average of 5% of the patients per month (as shown by rectal swabs taken at intervals throughout the trial, Fig. 1). In contrast, only one of 25 patients treated with nitrofurantoin macrocrystals and evaluable for this purpose demonstrated any nitrofurantoin-resistant *E. coli* at any time during the 12 months of treatment. The difference in the development of resistance to these antibiotics was sufficient to explain the better results using nitrofurantoin macrocrystals.

In a smaller trial (9), each of 15 women were randomized to receive single nightly doses of nitrofurantoin macrocrystals 100 mg, trimethoprim 100 mg, trimethoprim 40 mg/sulfamethoxazole 200 mg, or placebo. The patients in this trial were older, averaging 52 to 56 years. However, they did not have a greater incidence of radiologic abnormalities. All antibiotics were highly effective, with, as expected, poor results in the placebo-treated group (Table 5). All three regimens were well tolerated, with only one drug-related discontinuation due to a skin reaction in a patient treated with trimethoprim. Both trimethoprim and TMP-SMX partially eradicated *E. coli* from the rectal flora and did not select for resistance. However, colonization by enterococci of the urethral and vaginal areas was noted in patients receiving trimethoprim. We do not regard this as significant; in our experience enterococci are part of the normal flora of these areas (28).

Table 5 Comparative efficacy of low-dose, long-term therapy[a]

	Nitrofurantoin macrocrystals	Trimethoprim	Trimethoprim-sulfamethoxazole	Placebo
Number of evaluable patients	13	14	13	13
Number of patients with infections during low-dose, long-term therapy[b]	1	0	1	10
Number of infections per patient year	0.14	0	0.15	2.8

[a] Dosage schedule: nitrofurantoin macrocrystals, 100 mg, trimethoprim, 100 mg, or trimethoprim, 40 mg/sulfamethoxazole, 200 mg, nightly; [b] in each case of infection while on active treatment, symptoms and bacteriuria were present. (Data from reference 9.)

Table 6 Comparative efficacy of low-dose, long-term therapy with nitrofurantoin macrocrystals and norfloxacin[a]

	Nitrofurantoin macrocrystals	Norfloxacin
Number of evaluable patients	31	33
Total patient days of therapy	9755	10 930
Number of bacteriuric episodes while on therapy	3	3
Percent of patients with no bacteriuric episodes	90%	91%
Percent of patients with no symptomatic episodes	65%	70%

[a] Dosage schedule: nitrofurantoin macrocrystals, 100 mg, or norfloxacin, 200 mg, nightly. (Data from reference 10.)

The final trial reviewed here compared the efficacy and safety of nitrofurantoin macrocrystals and norfloxacin, a fluoroquinolone. Patients were treated with nightly doses of either nitrofurantoin macrocrystals, 100 mg, or norfloxacin, 200 mg. Equivalent efficacy (Table 6) was obtained in both groups. Only three patients in each group became infected while receiving preventive therapy. Each drug reduced the rate of infection 8.5-fold or greater, compared with the year preceding entry into the trial when patients were not receiving low-dose, long-term therapy. The frequency and severity of side effects were also similar; four patients treated with nitrofurantoin macrocrystals and six with norfloxacin discontinued therapy due to drug-related adverse reactions. Nitrofurantoin macrocrystals and norfloxacin were similarly safe and effective in this study (10).

EXPERIENCE WITH NITROFURANTOIN MACROCRYSTALS: SUMMARY AND CONCLUSIONS

During the course of the four trials reviewed above, 121 of the total patients evaluated were treated daily with 100 mg of nitrofurantoin, in most cases for one year. Between 59% and 92% of patients went through the entire study without experiencing symptoms of infections, despite pretreatment recurrence rates with a median of seven infections per year (10). (The 92% figure was obtained in the six-month trial (9).) Also, 88% to 92% of patients remained free of bacteriuria.

Resistance to nitrofurantoin was not acquired among strains of E. coli. Intrinsically resistant organisms such as Proteus sp in the fecal flora did not appear to increase, and these were not a source of infection (5). This can be attributed to nitrofurantoin macrocrystals apparently not altering the composition of the fecal flora.

All of these trials contained 20% to 28% of patients with radiologic abnormalities. Our findings show that these patients benefit from low-dose, long-term therapy as much as did patients without radiologic abnormalities. Several trials show that the efficacy of nitrofurantoin macrocrystals was clearly superior to that of methenamine salts. Nitrofurantoin macrocrystals is also superior to trimethoprim in an environment where trimethoprim resistance was relatively common (as in the United Kingdom). Under these circumstances recurrence was primarily due to breakthrough by trimethoprim-resistant E. coli strains. However, in studies in the United States and Canada (9,29,30) where the TMP-SMX resistance is considerably lower than in the United Kingdom, the low-dose, long-term efficacy of nitrofurantoin macrocrystals was equivalent to that of TMP-SMX. Interim analysis of an ongoing trial indicates that norfloxacin and macrocrystalline nitrofurantoin are equally effective (10).

In comparative trials versus methenamine hippurate and trimethoprim, nitrofurantoin was associated with a higher rate of drug-related side effects and discontinuation. The use of nitrofurantoin macrocrystals, instead of the microcrystalline form, would no doubt have reduced the rate of adverse effects in our first trial (31). The more frequent side effects observed with nitrofurantoin in the second trial must be balanced against the more frequent failure of treatment in the trimethoprim-treated group. No patients treated with nitrofurantoin macrocrystals discontinued the trials owing to lack of effectiveness. In the two other trials, there was no significant difference in the frequency of side effects during therapy with nitrofurantoin macrocrystals, trimethoprim, TMP-SMX, and norfloxacin.

It is not agreed by various workers whether the use of TMP-SMX for preventive therapy is preferable to trimethoprim alone (4).

Clearly, both combination therapy and monotherapy reduce the rate of infections compared with absence of treatment. It is not clear whether the presence of sulfonamide reduces the chance for trimethoprim resistance to emerge; more comparative studies are required to settle this question. The idiosyncratic and potentially severe side effects attributable to the sulfonamide component are also a problem (4). While these are rare in acute infections, they are naturally of increasing concern with long-term use. This fixed combination is not indicated in the United States for long-term suppressive or low-dose, long-term therapy (32).

Generally, long-term treatment with norfloxacin does not pose the problems cited above with TMP-SMX. However, the fluoroquinolones are contraindicated during pregnancy and lactation because of their possible adverse effects on developing cartilage and joint structure (as revealed by animal studies) (33). Therefore, before prescribing quinolones to women of childbearing age, the clinician must be sure that the patient is not pregnant and is using an effective means of birth control. This is especially important for long-term therapy.

In summary, in my experience, nitrofurantoin macrocrystals has been shown to be highly effective in low-dose, long-term preventive therapy, with a recommended dose of 100 mg nightly. Fivefold or greater reductions in the frequency of recurrence were obtained in all instances. Tolerance of nitrofurantoin macrocrystals can be a problem in the first month of treatment but is less so thereafter. As with any long-term drug regimen, nitrofurantoin therapy should be monitored by the patient's physician. Nitrofurantoin is not associated with the development of bacterial resistance in susceptible strains, such as *E. coli*, a particular advantage in long-term therapy. Nitrofurantoin macrocrystals is a cost-effective method of preventing recurrent urinary tract infection.

REFERENCES

(1) Corriere JN, Hanno PM, Hooton T, Snyder HM. Cystitis: Evolving standard of care. *Patient Care* 1988; **22**: 33-47.
(2) Schaeffer AJ. Recurrent urinary tract infection in the female patient. *Urology* 1988; **32** (suppl 3): 12-25.
(3) Brumfitt W, Smith GW, Hamilton-Miller JMT, Gargan RA. A clinical comparison between Macrodantin and trimethoprim for prophylaxis in women with recurrent urinary infections. *J Antimicrob Chemother* 1988; **16**: 111-120.
(4) Kasanen A, Sundquist H, Elo J, Anttila M, Kangas L. Secondary prevention of urinary tract infections. The role of trimethoprim alone. *Ann Clin Res* 1983; **15**: 1-36.
(5) Brumfitt W, Cooper J, Hamilton-Miller JMT. Prevention of recurrent urinary infections in women: a comparative trial between nitrofurantoin and methenamine hippurate. *J Urol* 1981; **126**: 71-74.
(6) Ormonde NW, Gray JA, Murdoch JM, et al. Chronic bacteriuria due to *Escherichia coli*. I. Assessment of the value of combined short- and long-term treatment with cycloserine, nitrofurantoin, and sulfadimidine. *J Infect Dis* 1969; **120**: 82-86.
(7) Bailey RR, Roberts AP, Gower PE, De Wardener HE. Prevention of urinary-tract infection with low-dose nitrofurantoin. *Lancet* 1971; **ii**: 1112-1114.
(8) Gow JG. A comparative trial of methenamine hippurate and hexamine mandelate in prevention of recurrent infection of the urinary tract. *Practitioner* 1974; **213**: 97-101.
(9) Stamm WE, Counts GW, Wagner KF, et al. Antimicrobial prophylaxis of recurrent urinary tract infections: a double-blind, placebo-controlled trial. *Ann Intern Med* 1980; **92**: 770-775.
(10) Brumfitt W, Hamilton-Miller JMT. Long-term prophylaxis of urinary infection: a clinical trial of norfloxacin versus Macrodantin (abstract). *2nd International symposium on new quinolones*, Geneva, Switzerland, August 1988.
(11) Iravani A. Bacterial infections of the urinary tract—female. In: Rakel RE, ed. *Conn's current therapy*. Philadelphia: WB Saunders, 1987: 538-541.
(12) Parsons CL. Lower urinary tract infections in women. *Urol Clin North Am* 1987; **14**: 247-250.
(13) Stamey TA: *Pathogens and treatment of urinary tract infections*. Baltimore: Williams & Wilkins Co, 1980.
(14) Grüneberg RN, Leigh DA, Brumfitt W. *Escherichia coli* serotypes in urinary tract infection: studies in domiciliary, antenatal and hospital practice. In: O'Grady FW, Brumfitt WD, eds. *Urinary tract infections*. London: Oxford University Press, 1968: 68-79.
(15) Brumfitt W, Gargan RA, Hamilton-Miller, JMT. Periurethral enterobacterial carriage preceding urinary infection. *Lancet* 1984; **i**: 824-826.
(16) Parsons CL, Schmidt JD. In vitro bacterial adherence to vaginal cells of normal and cystitis-prone women. *J Urol* 1980; **123**: 184-187.
(17) Schaeffer AJ, Jones JM, Dunn JK. Association of *in vitro Escherichia coli* adherence to vaginal and buccal epithelial cells with susceptibility of women to recurrent urinary tract infections. *N Engl J Med* 1981; **304**: 1062-1066.
(18) Landes RR. Long-term, low-dosage cinoxacin therapy for the prevention of recurrent urinary tract infections. *J Urol* 1980; **123**: 47-50.
(19) King LR, Kazmi SO, Belman AB. Natural history of vesicoureteral reflux: Outcome of a trial of nonoperative therapy. *Urol Clin North Am* 1974; **1**: 441-455.
(20) Govan DE, Fair WR, Friedland GW, Filly RA. Management of children with urinary tract infections: the Stanford experience. *Urology* 1975; **6**: 273-286.
(21) Brumfitt W, Condie AP. Urinary infection. In: Phillips EE, Barnes J, Newton M. *Scientific foundations of obstetrics and gynaecology*. 2nd ed. London: Heinemann Medical, 1977: 754-767.

(22) Freeman RB, Smith WMc, Richardson JA, et al. Long-term therapy for chronic bacteriuria in men: US Public Health Service cooperative study. Ann Intern Med 1975; 83: 133.
(23) Brumfitt W, Smith GW, Hamilton-Miller, JMT. Management of recurrent urinary infection: the place for a urinary infection clinic. In: Asscher AW, Brumfitt W, eds. *Microbial diseases in nephrology*. Chichester, England: John Wiley & Sons, 1986: 291–308.
(24) Brumfitt W, Hamilton-Miller JMT. The optimal duration of antibiotic treatment of urinary infections. In: Neu HC, Williams JD, eds. *New trends in urinary tract infections*. Basel, Switzerland: Karger, 1988: 62–77.
(25) Martinez FC, Kindrachuk RW, Thomas E, Stamey TA. Effect of prophylactic low dose cephalexin on fecal and vaginal bacteria. *J Urol* 1985; **133**: 994.
(26) Brumfitt W, Hamilton-Miller JMT. Recurrent urinary infections in women: clinical trial of cephradine as a prophylactic agent. *Infection* 1987; **15**: 344.
(27) Brumfitt W, Hamilton-Miller JMT. Changing role of cotrimoxazole in the treatment of recurrent urinary infections: a comparison with Augmentin. *Br J Clin Pract* 1985; **39**: 346.
(28) Cooper J, Brumfitt W, Hamilton-Miller JMT, Reynolds AV. The role of periurethral colonization in the aetiology of recurrent urinary infection in women. *Br J Obstet Gynaecol* 1980; **87**: 1145.
(29) Ronald AR, Harding GKM, Mathias R, Wong CK, Muir P. Prophylaxis of recurring urinary tract infection in females: a comparison of nitrofurantoin with trimethoprim-sulfamethoxazole. *Can Med Assoc J* 1975; **122**: 13s.
(30) Stamey TA, Condy M, Mihara G. Prophylactic efficacy of nitrofurantoin macrocrystals and trimethoprim-sulfamethoxazole in urinary infections. *N Engl J Med* 1977; **96**: 78.
(31) Hailey FJ, Glascock HW. Gastrointestinal intolerance to a new microcrystalline from of nitrofurantoin: a collaborative study. *Curr Ther Res* 1967; **9**: 600.
(32) *Physicians' desk reference* (PDR). 42nd ed. Oradell, NJ: Medical Economics Co, 1988.
(33) *British National Formulary No. 15*. London: British Medical Association, 1988: 220.

Special considerations in the management of acute urinary tract infection

P. E. V. Van Kerrebroeck

Department of Urology, Sint Radboud University Hospital, Geert Grooteplein, Nijmegen, The Netherlands

ABSTRACT

The treatment of complicated and uncomplicated urinary tract infections is reviewed, with an emphasis on diagnosis and morbidity. The primary cause of microbial invasion of the urinary tract is retrograde colonization by intestinal pathogens; other contributing factors include hormonal control of vaginal pH and length of the urethra. Most uncomplicated UTIs are caused by a single pathogen such as *Escherichia coli*. Findings at Sint Radboud University Hospital confirmed the preponderance of *E. coli* involvement, with *Klebsiella* and enterococci in second and third positions, respectively. University Hospital sensitivity data showed widespread resistance to many common antibacterials, particularly to amoxicillin and co-trimoxazole. Nitrofurantoin macrocrystals is a noted exception.

INTRODUCTION

Urinary tract infection (UTI) is a broad term used to indicate the presence of microorganisms in the urine and infection of the structures of the urinary tract, extending from the kidney to the urethral meatus and including adjacent organs such as the prostate.

Both diagnosis and treatment must make a distinction between uncomplicated and complicated infections. An uncomplicated UTI is one in which no structural or neurologic lesions are present. Whereas, complicated infections result when anatomic abnormalities or stones cause obstruction or when neurologic lesions interfere with urine drainage (1).

Important differences also exist between acute and chronic infections. Acute infections often mark the first episode of microbial invasion, are typical of the majority of UTIs, and generally respond well to antimicrobial therapy. The most common invading organism is *Escherichia coli*.

Chronic infections are those in which the urinary tract has been repeatedly invaded by bacteria, resulting in residual inflammation. Generally, chronic

---

Management of urinary tract infections, edited by Lloyd H. Harrison, 1990; Royal Society of Medicine Services International Congress and Symposium Series No. 154, published by Royal Society of Medicine Services Limited.

infections should be treated as complicated infections, because they often persist, despite antimicrobial therapy, until the obstruction is cleared or the voiding abnormality is corrected. The distinction between acute and chronic infection, however, is not always clear-cut. For example, acute exacerbations are possible in patients with chronic infection.

Infection may be expressed predominantly at a single site; the kidney (pyelonephritis); the bladder (cystitis); the prostate (prostatitis); or the urethra (urethritis). However, even if the infection is localized, one must remember the entire urinary tract is at risk of bacterial invasion.

UTIs may at times be limited to bacteria in the urine, and they may be asymptomatic. At other times infection may be characterized by an inflammatory response to microbial invasion of specific regions of the urinary tract. In either case, the presence of microorganisms is essential to the diagnosis, since noninfectious agents may also produce inflammation. Therefore, the concept of 'significant bacteriuria' has been developed, meaning that microorganisms are not only present in urine, but are in increasing concentration; these microorganisms may be derived from infected tissues. This concept differs from 'bacteriuria', which merely indicates the presence of bacteria in the urine regardless of the source. The distinction is important as urine can be contaminated, by surrounding tissues in women, or by simply passing through the urethra (in men and women).

MORBIDITY

UTIs have a significant impact on the general population. According to estimates, cystitis accounts for 1% of all office visits in the United States. Disorders of the genitourinary system account for 6.6% and respiratory conditions for 14.1% of all office visits. Although urologists in the United States treat about 23% of the patients with cystitis and 16% of those with pyelonephritis, these figures in other countries may vary (2).

Data from a health insurance company survey of 5835 people between the ages of 14 and 61 show a high incidence of UTIs. The overall rate was 12% in men and 43% in women. The women's rate was 37.8% in the 18 to 24 age-group, rising to 40% to 50% among those 25 and older. These data demonstrate the considerable morbidity associated with UTIs in otherwise healthy populations (3).

SYMPTOMS

The symptomatology of UTIs is variable and sometimes misleading. Clinical findings may suggest 'ordinary' cystitis, acute pyelonephritis, or even urosepsis (4). However, sometimes the only symptom is fever, or especially in children, gastrointestinal complaints (5,6). There can even be infection without symptoms. The severity of symptoms is not always related to the danger of underlying problems. Furthermore, the localization of symptoms does not always correlate with the localization of infection.

Acute cystitis comprises the majority of acute uncomplicated UTIs. It can cause bladder symptoms such as suprapubic pain or urethral burning. Sometimes the burning is constant; other times it is associated only with micturition usually at the end of voiding. Often urinary frequency persists throughout the night. Infection may be evident on macroscopic examination of the urine; urine may be grossly cloudy, malodorous, even bloody. Confirmation of infection, however, must be by microscopic urine examination.

Uncomplicated cystitis does not involve fever. If present, fever may be a sign of parenchymal invasion of the prostate or kidneys. Cystitis can cause hematuria without inflammation of other organs. At cystoscopy, the bladder mucosa will appear red and swollen, with signs of inflammation. Submucosal bleeding and mucosal ulcerations may be apparent. These findings may be localized throughout the bladder or limited to the trigone.

The prognosis for uncomplicated cystitis is favorable; with proper treatment symptoms disappear after two or three days. All too often, however, patients discontinue treatment as soon as symptomatic relief is achieved (typically between the third and fourth day of therapy) but before the infection is completely eradicated. This may be the biggest reason for recurrent infection.

CLINICAL PROBLEMS

In children younger than one year, the incidence of UTI is about 2% to 3%. In this age-group, UTI is the most important bacterial problem after respiratory tract infection. Infection occurs four times more frequently in boys than in girls. As the female anatomy favors UTI, this frequency indicates that underlying disease is often the cause of infection in boys. At the age of 1 year, the incidence is approximately 1%, and the rate of infection is equal in boys and girls. However, beyond this age, frequency in girls rises to about 1.6%, and in boys declines to 0.3% (7,8).

With the onset of sexual activity, the incidence of UTIs in females increases to about 4%. By the beginning of menopause, UTI frequency reaches 10%; it climbs to 15% for women 65 and older. In men, the incidence of UTIs remains at 1% for those under 65 and elevates to about 3.5% for those who are older. These statistics are merely indicative as they are affected by methods of diagnosis used and the UTI classification system followed.

PATHOGENESIS

The primary site of UTI can be parenchymal with secondary contamination occurring throughout the urinary tract and the urine. More often, infection begins as a microbial invasion of the urinary tract that evolves into parenchymal infection. Most UTIs occur because of retrograde bacterial colonization, which is the reason for the prevalence of cystitis and other lower urinary tract infections (LUTIs) in women. This also explains why most pathogens are gram-negative and intestinal in origin. Sometimes the saprophytic floras of the perineum or anterior urethra are responsible; these pathogens are mostly gram-positive.

Under normal circumstances, urine should be sterile. Because the composition of urine is favorable to bacterial invasion, certain defense mechanisms are built in to limit bacterial penetration. Infection will occur only when these defense mechanisms are disturbed. In women, penetration of bacteria is limited due to growth inhibition in the anterior vagina. This is influenced by the vaginal pH, which is in turn controlled by hormones (estrogens). In men, the length of the urethra is itself a limiting factor.

The bladder has its own defenses, which include mechanical, antibacterial, and immunologic mechanisms.

Mechanical

Regular voiding without residual urine is essential. Voiding clears the bladder and limits bacterial proliferation. With stasis, the bladder bacterial count could theoretically double every 45 min. Production of 1.5 to 2 l of urine a day results in sufficient dilution of urine and limits bacteriuria. Finally, the integrity of bladder mucosa is essential. Each mucosal lesion is a site for bacterial fixation and growth and can interfere with the antibacterial and immunologic functions of the bladder.

Antibacterial

In the normal bladder, less than 10% of residual bacteria will survive after 4 h. The exact mechanism of this bactericidal activity remains unexplained.

Immunologic

Small amounts of immunoglobulins have been found in bladder urine. Their specific role in immune defense is unknown (9).

Clearly, whenever these defense mechanisms are not effective, infection can occur. Recent research also suggests genetic predisposition may play a role in UTIs. Genetic differences at the cellular level may influence bacterial adherence, making certain individuals, usually women, more prone to UTIs (10). Such is the case whenever voiding is disturbed. Therefore, an analysis of individual micturition behaviour is essential in determining the pathogenesis of UTI.

Additionally, the role of sexual activity in UTIs is generally acknowledged (1,11). Quantitative research has shown that UTI is four to 10 times less frequent in nuns than in the general female population between the ages of 15 and 35 (12). The issue is controversial. Possibly, sexual intercourse displaces the urethral meatus, which leads to vaginovesical reflux, vaginal contamination, and translocation of saprophytic flora.

PATHOGENS

Most UTIs are caused by gram-negative organisms. The presence of typical enteric flora in UTIs suggests an ascending infection. Uncomplicated infections most often result from a single bacterial species. Enterobacteriaceae are the most commonly encountered organisms. In about 80% of LUTIs, *E. coli* is the causative organism. In young women in outpatient settings, gram-positive *Staphylococcus saprophyticus* is the second most common organism, accounting for about 10% to 15% of infections (13). Its presence on the skin suggests it as the possible source of infection (4,14).

Other gram-negative bacteria such as *Proteus* and *Pseudomonas* are seldom found in acute UTIs in the general population (4,14). When found, they raise suspicions about underlying disease. These are more commonly found in hospital-acquired infections (Table 1).

Hospital-acquired UTIs are, for the most part, complicated, because of the underlying illness of the patient (urologic or otherwise), instrumentation, or the uropathogens encountered. These uropathogens show marked antimicrobial resistance.

Table 1 Most common isolates from hospitalized patients with urinary tract infections[a]

Microorganism	%
Escherichia coli	31.7
Enterococci	14.9
Pseudomonas aeruginosa	12.5
Klebsiella sp	7.6
Proteus sp	7.3
Candida sp	5.1
Enterobacter sp	4.4
Coagulase-negative staphylococci	3.7
Other fungi	2.0
Staphylococcus aureus	1.6
Citrobacter sp	1.4
Serratia sp	1.2
Group B streptococci	1.0
Bacteroides and other anaerobes	0.0
All others	5.6

[a] These data are based on 13 165 isolates from urine. (Data from reference 24.)

PROBLEMS WITH RESISTANT ORGANISMS

A microbiologic survey was conducted in Sint Radboud University Hospital during three months of 1988. Uropathogens from 244 outpatients with uncomplicated UTI were cultured. Of the pathogens identified (Table 2): *E. coli* was isolated in 112 cases, *Klebsiella* in 22, and enterococcus in 21. Among the two most prevalent pathogens, diverse resistance was noted (Table 3).

Twenty-eight percent of the *E. coli* infections exhibited resistance to amoxicillin and 22% were resistant to co-trimoxazole. Of the *Klebsiella* infections, 100% exhibited resistance to amoxicillin and 4% to co-trimoxazole. Nitrofurantoin was effective against 87% of the *Klebsiella* infections and 92% of the *E. coli* infections. Pipemidic acid and ciprofloxacin, a recently introduced antibiotic, demonstrated the

Table 2 Pathogenesis of acute uncomplicated urinary tract infection[a]

Pathogen	No.
Escherichia coli	112
Klebsiella	22
Enterococci	21
Proteus sp	1
Coagulase-negative staphylococci	16
Coagulase-positive staphylococci	10
Enterobacter	13
Pseudomonas aeruginosa	8
Other	24
Total	244

[a] Infections studied in urologic outpatient department of Sint Radboud University Hospital, June through August 1988.
Source: Unpublished results of I. Breuker, A. Horrevorts, P. Van Kerrebroeck, Sint Radboud University Hospital, 1988.

Table 3 Resistance of pathogens[a]

	% resistant	
	Escherichia coli ($n=112$)[b]	Klebsiella ($n=22$)[b]
Amoxicillin	28	100
Co-trimoxazole	22	4
Nitrofurantoin	8	13
Pipemidic acid	3	13
Ciprofloxacin	0	4

[a] Infections studied in urologic outpatient department of Sint Radboud University Hospital, June through August 1988; [b] n = number of isolates.
Source: Unpublished results of I. Breuker, A. Horrevorts, P. Van Kerrebroeck, Sint Radboud University Hospital, 1988.

Table 4 Sensitivity of pathogens[a]

	% Sensitivity	
	Escherichia coli ($n=452$)	Klebsiella ($n=96$)
Amoxicillin	74	7
Co-trimoxazole	84	92
Nitrofurantoin	91	60
Pipemidic acid	97	83
Ciprofloxacin	100	93

[a] Infections studied in Sint Radboud University Hospital, January through September 1987.

Table 5 Antibiotics prescribed in general practice and sensitivity of uropathogens[a]

	Sensitivity (%)			
	Escherichia coli	Klebsiella[b]	Streptococcus faecalis[b]	Proteus[b]
Amoxicillin	70 (834)	2 (200)	99 (241)	69 (263)
Cefazolin	91 (834)	91 (200)	25 (241)	77 (263)
Tetracycline	70 (834)	94 (200)	43 (240)	16 (263)
Sulfonamide	61 (636)	85 (136)	0 (128)	83 (168)
Trimethoprim	77 (629)	82 (134)	86 (127)	82 (182)
Nitrofurantoin	97 (629)	87 (134)	99 (127)	14 (168)
Pipemidic acid	98 (629)	90 (134)	0 (127)	98 (168)

[a] Data was acquired in The Netherlands during January 1982 to June 1988; [b] Numbers in parentheses represent total numbers of strains tested.
Source: Sabbe L, Goudswaard J, Hendrickx B, Stichting Streeklaboratorium Zeeland, Goies, The Netherlands, unpublished data.

least resistance overall. When these sensitivities are compared with data from nine months in 1987 for the entire hospital (Table 4), resistance to nitrofurantoin remained at about the same low level for *E. coli* and at a reasonable level for *Klebsiella*. Data from the community also confirm the continued activity of nitrofurantoin (Table 5).

DIAGNOSTIC PROBLEMS

Diagnostically, the distinction between uncomplicated and complicated infections is most important. It is a particularly useful guide to prognosis and response to therapy. As mentioned earlier, an uncomplicated infection occurs most often in an otherwise healthy woman with a normal urinary tract. Other important considerations include the patient's age, sex, and renal function. In addition, note specific medical conditions such as pregnancy and diabetes.

The first step is to confirm the diagnosis. The most simple, rapid, and cost-effective diagnostic procedure is microscopic examination of clean, freshly voided urine to determine the presence of bacteria and leukocytes. However, the results are not always conclusive. Bacteria may not be visible microscopically despite significant concentrations, and contaminating vaginal flora may mimic infecting bacteria. Also pyuria (10 or more leukocytes per high-power field) may possibly result from inflammatory disorders other than infection.

Because of these diagnostic difficulties, quantitative urine culture provides the most accurate assessment of the bacteriologic status of bladder urine. Urine that was actually sterile in the bladder will contain either no bacteria or a small number of contaminants, colony forming units (CFUs) less than 10 000/ml. 'Significant bacteriuria' means CFUs are greater than 100 000/ml (4). This is the traditional criterion, and 60% to 86% of cultures from patients with UTIs contain CFUs greater than or equal to 1 000 000/ml.

Significant bacteriuria is a laboratory test result, not a disease. The clinician must take into account the patient's medical history and current health. A low-count UTI may be clinically significant or just an abnormal finding. Strictly speaking, asymptomatic bacteriuria cannot be considered an infection if pyuria is not present. This will be the case in about 50% of infections (1,13).

THERAPY

The goal of antimicrobial therapy in uncomplicated UTIs is to reduce or eliminate morbidity and prevent symptomatic infections. Therefore, when the diagnosis of UTI is made, even if the infection is uncomplicated, antimicrobial therapy must be initiated. Along with antibiotics, the physician should give the patient practical advice on how to avoid recurrent infections. Elimination of asymptomatic bacteriuria is desirable, but not essential, in all cases.

The choice of drug depends upon the severity of the infection, the sensitivity of the organism to a specific agent, ease of administration, risk of side effects, and relative cost (15). As nearly 90% of uncomplicated UTIs are caused by *E. coli*, which is susceptible to most oral antimicrobial agents, the choice is wide. However, drug selection must be based mainly on relative expense and toxicity.

In 10% to 15% of females with uncomplicated infections, *Staph. saprophyticus* is the vector. In my opinion, nitrofurantoin macrocrystals is effective against both *E. coli* and *S. saprophyticus* and has proven valuable for the majority of uncomplicated infections. Moreover, organisms continue to remain sensitive. This is probably because of the difficulty enteric bacteria have in developing resistance, and because only about 2% of nitrofurantoin is excreted in the feces (16). Within 24–48 h, urine should be rendered sterile. If not, the treatment should be considered a failure and the drug should be changed. How long to treat uncomplicated infections still remains a point for discussion (15,17). The major problem in uncomplicated infections is the high rate of recurrence (up to 80%

within one year). However, most recurrences in uncomplicated infections in women will be due to infection with a new organism (species or type) rather than to relapses with the same organism (18).

If one could be sure an infection is really uncomplicated, shorter courses of therapy would be possible. For example, pure bladder bacteriuria could be eliminated by single-dose therapy with an effective agent, keeping in mind the diagnostic problems UTIs can present. The optimum duration of therapy depends upon a thorough knowledge of the patient's history and the clinical assessment. In uncomplicated infections, therapy usually lasts up to 14 days. Interestingly, most trials indicate 10 days of therapy are as effective as two weeks (19). Several studies, however, suggest a three-day course of therapy may be effective for some patients (19-21). Few researchers have made comparative studies of three-day versus 10-day courses (22,23). In our observation, the relapse rate has been higher with three-day therapies. In our department we continue to prescribe the 10-day treatment for most patients with uncomplicated infections.

PATIENT COMPLIANCE

To achieve satisfactory compliance, we explain to our patients in a straightforward fashion their medical problem, what they should and should not do during treatment, and what precautions can be taken to prevent recurrent infections. We stress the importance of completing the entire course of antibiotic therapy and correct voiding hygiene. We recommend drinking one and one-half to two liters of water daily in addition to their normal intake to force diuresis. We instruct patients to make a conscious effort to void frequently and completely in order to prevent the buildup of bladder bacteria (1). Patients are advised to void before and after sexual intercourse. They are counselled on perineal hygiene—front to back. Only through appropriate therapy, along with patient education and compliance, will patients and their physicians achieve satisfying results in managing acute uncomplicated UTIs.

REFERENCES

(1) Hanno PM. Etiology of cystitis: factors affecting management strategies. *Fam Pract Recert* 1987; **9S**: 14.

(2) National Center for Health Statistics. *Vital and health statistics of the National Center for Health Statistics*, October 12, 1977.

(3) Kunin CM. *Detection, prevention and management of urinary tract infection*. Philadelphia: Lea & Febiger, 1987.

(4) Corriere JN, Hanno PM, Hooton T, Snyder HM. Cystitis: evolving standard of care. *Patient Care* 1988; **22**: 33–47.

(5) Bollgren I. UTI in children and adolescents. *Contemp Obstet Gynecol* 1986; **27**: 167.

(6) Dossett JH. Management of urinary tract infections in children and adolescents: preventing complications. *Fam Pract Recert* 1987; **9S**: 21.

(7) Fiveash JG Jr, Foster EA, Paquin AJ Jr. Antibody response in lower urinary tract infection. *J Urol* 1964; **92(5)**: 545–548.

(8) Kass EH. Bacteriuria and the diagnosis of infections of the urinary tract. *Arch Intern Med* 1957; **100**: 709–714.

(9) Uehling DT. Future approaches to the management of urinary tract infections. *Urol Clin North Am* 1986; **13**: 749–758.

(10) Andriole VT. Urinary tract infections: recent developments. *J Infect Dis* 1987; **156**: 865–869.

(11) McCaskey GM. Choosing therapy for acute urinary tract infection in the sexually active woman—a case presentation. *Fam Pract Recert* 1987; **8S**: 51.
(12) Kunin CM, McCormack RC. An epidemiologic study of bacteriuria and blood pressure among nuns and working women. *N Engl J Med* 1968; **278**: 635–642.
(13) Stamm WE. Prevention of urinary tract infections. *Am J Med* 1984; **76S**: 148–154.
(14) Duff P. Urinary tract infections in pregnant women. *Fam Pract Recert* 1987; **9S**: 27.
(15) Parsons CL. Protocol for treatment of typical urinary tract infections: criteria for antimicrobial selection. *Urology* 1988; **32S**: 22–27.
(16) D'Arcy PF. Nitrofurantoin. *Drug Intell Clin Pharm* 1985; **19**: 540–547.
(17) Parsons CL. Antibiotic selection for lower urinary tract infections. *Fam Pract Recert* 1987; **9S**: 9.
(18) Stamey TA. *Pathogenesis and treatment of urinary tract infections*. Baltimore: Williams & Wilkins Co., 1980; **4**: 122.
(19) Charlton CA, Crowther A, Davees JJ, et al. Three-day to 10-day chemotherapy for urinary tract infection in general practice. *Br Med J* 1976; **1**: 124–6.
(20) Faer WR, Crane DB, Peterson LJ, et al. Three-day treatment of urinary tract infection. *J Urol* 1980; **123**: 717–21.
(21) Grüneberg RN, Reely PM, Luppen KL, et al. A randomized study of single-dose, three-day, and seven-day treatment of cystitis in women. *J Infect Dis* 1986; **153**: 277–282.
(22) Liedtke RK, Ebel S, Missler B, Stein L. Single-dose pharmacokinetics of macrocrystalline nitrofurantoin formulations. *Arzneimittelforschung* 1980; **30** (pt 1): 833–836.
(23) Lohr JA, Hayden GF, Kesler RW, et al. Three-day therapy of lower urinary tract infections with nitrofurantoin: a randomized clinical trial. *J Pediatr* 1981; **99**: 980–983.
(24) Jarvis WR, White JM, Munn VP, et al. Nosocomial infections surveillance 1983. *MMWR* 1985; **33**: 14SS.

Managing recurrent urinary tract infections

S. G. Mulholland

Department of Urology, Thomas Jefferson University Medical College, Philadelphia, Pennsylvania, USA

ABSTRACT

To manage recurrent urinary tract infections (UTIs) appropriately, they must be evaluated in context. In infants and male patients, a recurrent UTI suggests an underlying anatomic anomaly. In contrast, recurrences in adult women are usually uncomplicated, acute infections. Microscopic analysis and dipstick testing suffice to diagnose the infection with most patients, but further evaluation may be necessary in specific instances. Self-medication with an appropriate antimicrobial may be a useful approach for patients who have multiple recurrences of uncomplicated UTI.

INTRODUCTION

To avoid possible confusion, basic terminology should be agreed upon before discussing urinary tract infections (UTIs). Various classification systems have been used to define UTI, which, for purposes of discussion, is taken to mean microbial invasion of any tissue of the urinary tract. The classic terminology divides these infections into acute, recurrent, relapsing, and chronic UTIs. However, these do not include the situation in which microbes are present in the urine without eliciting a classic infectious response. To describe this situation, some authors prefer the term asymptomatic bacteriuria or bacteriuria not associated with pyuria.

Other authors have tried to improve upon this classification system. Stamey devised more precise terms: first infections, unresolved bacteriuria, reinfections, and bacterial persistence [1]. These four basic categories may be subdivided into more descriptive smaller groups, such as male, female, hospital, community, uncomplicated, complicated, upper, and lower. More descriptive terminology can help the clinician manage the individual patient. For example, a typical case might be described as: a recurrent, female, community, uncomplicated lower urinary tract infection.

CLARIFYING THE TERMINOLOGY

A more complete description of the various kinds of UTIs encountered may clarify how the terminology can be used in practice. An acute infection occurs as a solitary event, with no relationship to any other infection or infecting organism. Usually, it is separated from other events by at least two or three months.

A recurrent infection is a series of infections, caused by different organisms or different serotypes and separated by at least three or four weeks. This term is synonymous with the term reinfection. Stamey refers to unresolved bacteriuria, which may have a variety of causes. These include: a resistant organism, development of resistance in an individual patient, multiple species with different sensitivities, azotemia, papillary necrosis, or staghorn calculus. Relapsing infection implies persistent infection by the organism that caused the original infection. This term most closely parallels Stamey's term 'bacterial persistence', which, in fact, describes an uncommon situation. Recurrent UTI with a new and different organism is far more common (2).

A chronic infection may be caused by one or more organisms and does not resolve with any form of treatment. It may be associated with some medical complicating factor, either at a distant site or from a site within the urinary tract.

INCIDENCE OF INFECTION

A number of factors may affect the incidence of infection. The age at which an infection occurs is important. The incidence of UTI in males exceeds that in females only during the neonatal period. Infections that occur in male infants, particularly premature, sick babies, are related to intrinsic urinary tract disease or to metastasis of bacteria from another part of the body, such as the lung (3–6).

After the neonatal period, the incidence of UTI in men decreases almost to zero. Beyond age 40, however, the incidence tends to rise. This is caused by developing intrinsic urinary tract disease or complicating medical diseases. The finding of a bacterial UTI in any man should alert the clinician to search for a pathologic cause.

In females, the incidence of UTI varies markedly at different ages (7). Probably the most important age-group in females with UTIs is children less than 1 year old. At this age, there is a high incidence of urinary tract disease—reflux or obstruction—and the renal scarring, which will be seen throughout life, occurs.

Also, with the initial presentation of UTI among girls in preschool and in the lower grades, a decrease in the incidence of urinary tract disorders is seen with advancing age (8,9). Girls who have had childhood bacteriuria are more likely to develop UTI as adults. In these cases, the relationship between bacteriuria and UTIs seems to be associated with some defect in the defense mechanism. After a relatively symptom-free period between the ages of 10 and 15, the incidence of UTIs then begins to increase again, presumably associated with sexual activity and pregnancy. Among other possible causative factors noted in the literature are oral and barrier contraceptives, menstruation, tampons, socioeconomics, hygiene, clothing, and diet (10).

The incidence of bacteriuria increases gradually—from 1% to 2% per decade—reaching 10% among postmenopausal women between the ages of 55 and 65 (11). Although the reason for this increase is not known, it probably is associated with a decrease in hormonal levels and vaginal antibacterial defense mechanisms. The latter decrease facilitates the bacterial entrance and colonization in the urinary tract.

Large-scale studies of women of childbearing age report that 4% to 6% are bacteriuric at any given time: Adult women account for about 30% of cases of symptomatic UTI. Women who are found to be bacteriuric through screening are seven times more likely to develop a symptomatic infection than are those whose urine cultures are free of organisms (12). Some 20% of all adult women will develop a UTI in their lifetimes, and between 3% and 5% of them will experience recurrent infections (11). According to one study, 28% of patients with a first acute infection will develop a recurrence within 18 months. With a second recurrence, 80% will develop another infection (13). There seems to be a population of women who have a propensity to develop recurrent UTIs (10–14). Recurrences are more likely in a patient who has a history of UTIs.

In adult women, most recurrences are acute, uncomplicated reinfections separated by relatively long periods of time; they should be treated in the same way the initial infections were treated. With no extenuating circumstances, one can assume that recurrences are not due to resistant or unusual pathogens. In women who have recurrences close together (two to four weeks), there is greater exposure to antimicrobials and therefore a good chance for flora changes and development of resistant organisms. Women who have recurrent infections often have prolonged infection-free intervals, and the reinfections tend to occur in clusters (15). It is important to remember this phenomenon when planning treatment strategies for recurrent UTIs.

WHO AND HOW TO EVALUATE

Which patients should be evaluated for possible UTIs has always been a matter of controversy. We are dealing with literally millions of patients, and guidelines are needed to help decide which might have significant disease. The following types of patients should be evaluated: males with bacterial infection; symptomatic girls less than 10 years of age; adults with a childhood history of UTI; and patients with recurrent or multiple infections, pyelonephritis, unusual organisms, poor clinical response, or persistent hematuria. Individuals with these signs and risk factors could have significant disease that may need surgical treatment and close follow-up.

The procedure for evaluating these patients has certainly changed in the past five or six years. Identification of the organism and antimicrobial sensitivity tests are necessary in individuals who have multiple recurrent infections or infections that are difficult to treat. Routine intravenous pyelograms (IVPs) are virtually obsolete in evaluating children and most adults. Probably, ultrasonic evaluation of the upper tracts and ureters is adequate for most patients. Only if the patient has hematuria or some other reason to outline the collecting systems carefully is there any need for IVP.

Cystoscopy, a procedure that was commonplace in the past, has added very little to diagnostic accuracy either in children or adults (16,17). Obviously, if there is some reason for direct observation of the urethra or bladder, such as hematuria, suspicion of cancer, or calculi, a cystoscopy might be indicated. In a child, a voiding cystourethrogram is a critical part of the evaluation. This test has been used less frequently in adults, because of the low yield of useful results. If the ultrasonic evaluation of an adult's upper tract and ureters is normal, a cystogram usually adds very little information. Urodynamic studies are indicated when the clinician suspects some neurologic abnormality.

MAKING THE DIAGNOSIS

In diagnosing a recurrent or a symptomatic UTI, the physician must determine which women who have acute symptoms of bacterial cystitis actually have the disease. While bacterial cystitis is the leading cause of UTIs, approximately one third of those who have acute symptoms have either sterile urine or some other cause for the symptoms (18). Other potential causes include sexually transmitted pathogens, such as *Chlamydia*, herpes, and *Trichomonas;* interstitial cystitis; carcinoma; calculi; or obstruction. In a recent large trial of empiric therapy for UTI in the United Kingdom, enrollment on the basis of symptoms alone produced a 31% incidence of false-positive treatment results for UTI (19).

In the past, a culture was obtained by the clean catch technique, but this method often resulted in contamination from the urethra and vagina. The more reliable clean catheterization or needle aspiration of the bladder has produced much more accurate information about bacterial counts and pyuria. The old theory that a bonafide UTI required a bacteria count greater than 10^5/ml has been seriously challenged recently. Counts below 10^5/ml have been demonstrated in between 20% and 50% of patients with documented UTIs. In patients with acute symptoms of cystitis, Kunz found 27% with counts of less than 10^4/ml (20). In studies of the acute dysuria syndrome, Stamm found that 47% of patients with UTIs had counts below 10^5/ml and 30% had counts of less than 10^4/ml (21). Thus, if one uses needle aspiration or clean catheterization, a count of greater than 10^2/ml probably indicates the patient's symptoms are caused by bladder bacteria. If the patient also has pyuria, almost assuredly the diagnosis is bacterial cystitis.

In about 80% of patients with bacterial infections, an in-office microscopic evaluation is sufficient to make an accurate diagnosis. Dipsticks that measure the transformation of nitrites to nitrates or measure levels of leukocyte esterase are about 80% accurate. A combination of the dipstick test and microscopic analysis probably achieves an accuracy of better than 80%. Infection is likely when the bacterial count is greater than 10^2/ml or when there is pyuria. However, a culture may be necessary in patients who have acute symptoms but whose counts are so low that bacteria are not seen microscopically. When a patient has multiple recurrent infections, or an infection that has been difficult to treat, identification of the organism and its antimicrobial sensitivities may be necessary.

MANAGING RECURRENT UTI

The management of patients' recurrent UTIs depends to a great extent on individual circumstances. In certain patients, repeated UTIs will lead to renal deterioration, but, fortunately, this is rare. However, those who have a childhood history of UTI, followed by pyelonephritis and scarring, are at risk for deterioration with repeated infections. Others who are at risk include individuals with residual urine, obstruction, neurologic disorders, reflux, calculus disease, and those with various metabolic, hematologic, and vascular medical problems. Identification of these special patients is very important so they can be followed closely.

Fortunately, most patients, especially females, who have recurrent UTIs have normal kidneys and urinary tracts, and their infections are not associated with urologic disease. Treatment is directed simply to sterilizing the urine and relieving the patients' symptoms. Most such patients can be followed up less closely.

The majority of UTIs are classified as recurrent, autoinfected, community, female infections. They are relatively easy to treat and control. The initial management goal, sterilization of the urine, can be achieved after a few days of therapy with a suitable antimicrobial agent. In fact, sterilization of the urine by short course therapy can be a method of differentiating simple from complicated UTI. A patient who does not respond to a short course of therapy may have a condition that is a cause of continual bacterial seeding, e.g., chronic pyelonephritis, stone disease, or prostatitis. If the patient continues to develop recurrent UTIs, I recommend short courses of treatment by self-medication with agents such as nitrofurantoin macrocrystals, norfloxacin, or trimethoprim-sulfamethoxazole (TMP-SMX) until urine is sterile.

Intermittent therapy with antimicrobials may possibly expose fecal flora to drug concentrations near their minimum inhibitory levels. Consequently, antimicrobials that are well absorbed in the upper gastrointestinal tract and low doses for more chronic treatment periods must be utilized to obviate changing flora and the development of resistance. Nitrofurantoin macrocrystals is an excellent choice because it does not foster resistance development (22,23).

Selection of the right medication for chronic therapy is important. The antibiotic must be well tolerated and low in cost; it must not develop resistance. It must have a good antimicrobial spectrum and have little effect on large-bowel flora. Patients who have vaginal colonization with potential urinary tract pathogens may benefit from antimicrobials that are excreted in the vaginal secretions. The antimicrobial we use most often for chronic treatment at bedtime or for self-medication is nitrofurantoin macrocrystals. Cephalexin, trimethoprim, TMP-SMX, or cinozacin may be utilized in short course therapy or in low-dose chronic therapy. Generally, these are reserved as backup therapy because of their potentially deleterious effect on fecal and vaginal flora. However, as mentioned above, these antimicrobials all seem to have the qualities necessary for either chronic therapy or self-medication.

If reinfection occurs, I instruct my patients to self-medicate by taking an antimicrobial for two days when they feel the onset of symptoms. If the symptoms seem to be recurring as often as once a month, I recommend daily medication or medication every other night for a six- to eight-week period. The drug can then be withdrawn and the patient observed. Cultures of each infection with sensitivity tests are unnecessary.

Usually, patients can be maintained on self-medication for long periods, provided they have been well educated about their infections. They report each infection to the office staff and are seen yearly. This regimen reduces the patient's visits to the hospital or doctor's office and subsequent expense (23).

Should any complications arise such as fever or flank pain, the patient is instructed to call the office immediately. If there appears to be some specific cause for the infections, such as menstruation or sexual activity, the patient may need medication only during these vulnerable periods.

CONCLUSION

Management of recurrent UTIs can be quite successful if one understands certain basic principles, such as whom to evaluate and the relationship of age to incidence. Evaluation and follow-up of these patients varies according to the classification of their infections. Our approach to this common clinical problem has changed considerably over the past decade, with the use of IVP and cystoscopy becoming nearly obsolete.

REFERENCES

(1) Stamey TA. A clinical classification of urinary tract infections based upon origin. *South Med J* 1975; **68**: 934–939.

(2) Stamey TA. Urinary tract infections in women. In: Stamey TA, ed. *Pathogenesis and treatment of urinary tract infections.* Baltimore: Williams and Wilkins Co., 1980; **4**: 122-209.
(3) Ginsburg CM, McCracken GH Jr. Urinary tract infections in young infants. *Pediatrics* 1982; **69**: 409-412.
(4) Bergström T, Larson H, Lincoln K, Winberg J. Studies of urinary tract infection in infancy and childhood: XII. Eighty consecutive patients with neonatal infection. *J Pediatr* 1972; **80**: 858-866.
(5) Drew JH, Acton CM. Radiological findings in newborn infants with urinary infection. *Arch Dis Child* 1976; **51**: 628-630.
(6) Littlewood JM. Sixty-six infants with urinary tract infection in the first month of life. *Arch Dis Child* 1972; **47**: 218-226.
(7) Stamey TA. Urinary tract infections in the female: a perspective. In: Remington JS, Swartz MN, eds. *Current clinical topics in infectious diseases.* New York: McGraw-Hill Book Company, 1981: 31-53.
(8) Kunin CM, Deutscher R, Paquin AJ. Urinary tract infection in school children: epidemiologic, clinical, and laboratory study. *Medicine* 1964; **43**: 91-130.
(9) Kunin CM, Zacha E, Paquin AJ. Urinary tract infections in school children. I. Prevalence of bacteriuria and associated urologic findings. *N Engl J Med* 1962; **266**: 1287-1296.
(10) Kunin CM. The concepts of "significant bacteriuria" and asymptomatic bacteriuria, clinical syndromes and the epidemiology of urinary tract infections. In: Kunin CM, ed. *Detection, prevention, and management of urinary tract infections.* 4th ed. Philadelphia: Lea & Febiger, 1987: chap 2.
(11) Kass EH, Savage WD, Santamarina BAG. The significance of bacteriuria in preventive medicine. In: Kass EH, ed. *Progress in pyelonephritis.* Philadelphia: FA Davis, 1964; **1**: 3.
(12) Gaymans R, Haverkorn MJ, Valkenberg HA, Goslings WR. A prospective study of urinary tract infections in a Dutch general practice. *Lancet* 1976; **ii**: 674-677.
(13) Harrison WO, Holmes KK, Belding ME, Wiesner PJ, Turck M. A prospective evaluation of recurrent urinary tract infection in women. *Clin Res* 1974; **22**: 125A.
(14) Stamey TA. The role of introital bacteria in recurrent urinary infections. *J Urol* 1973; **109**: 467-472.
(15) Kraft JK, Stamey TA. The natural history of symptomatic recurrent bacteriuria in women. *Medicine* 1977; **56**: 55-60.
(16) Engel G, Schaeffer AJ, Grayhack JT, Wendel EF. The role of excretory urography and cystoscopy in the evaluation and management of women with recurrent urinary tract infection. *J Urol* 1980; **123**: 190-191.
(17) Corriere JN Jr. Avoiding "overkill" in diagnosis and treatment of lower urinary tract infections. *Urology* 1988; **32** (suppl): 17-19.
(18) Johnson JR, Stamm WE. Diagnosis and treatment of acute urinary tract infections. *Infect Dis Clin North Am* 1987; **1**: 773-791.
(19) Pfau A, Sacks TG. An evaluation of midstream urine cultures in the diagnosis of urinary tract infections in females. *Urol Int* 1970; **25**: 326-341.
(20) Kunz HH, Sieberth HG, Freiberg J, Pulverer G, Schneider FJ. Zur Bedeutung der Blasenpunktion fur den sicheren Nachweis einer Bakteriurie. *Dtsch Med Wochenschr* 1975; **100**: 2252-2256, 2261-2264.
(21) Stamm WE, Wagner KF, Amsel R, *et al.* Causes of the acute urethral syndrome in women. *N Engl J Med* 1980; **303**: 409-415.
(22) Harding GKM, Ronald AR, Nicolle LE, *et al.* Long-term antimicrobial prophylaxis for recurrent urinary tract infection in women. *Rev Infect Dis* 1982; **4**: 438-443.
(23) Cunha BA: Nitrofurantoin: current concepts. *Urology* 1988; **32**: 67-71.

Special considerations in the management of complicated urinary tract infections

J. C. Nickel

Department of Urology, Queen's University, Kingston, Ontario, Canada

ABSTRACT

The majority of urinary tract infections (UTIs) occur in patients without apparent structural abnormalities of the urinary tract. These uncomplicated infections are usually easily treated with traditional antibiotic therapy. Unlike simple UTI, complicated UTI may result from four types of structural or acquired abnormalities of the urinary tract. These include: anomalies causing obstruction, stasis, or reflux; presence of foreign bodies such as a urinary catheter; infected urinary stones; and disorders allowing bacterial persistence within the urinary tract. Rational treatment should be based on an understanding of the pathogenic mechanisms that cause these complicated infections. Case reports of recurrent childhood UTI, catheter-associated nosocomial infections, struvite calculi, and chronic bacterial prostatitis are used to illustrate UTI management techniques, including surgical procedures and long-term antibiotic therapy.

INTRODUCTION

The treatment of urinary tract infection (UTI) requires an awareness of the interactions between host susceptibility and pathogen virulence factors in the development and persistence of these infections. The majority of UTIs occur in patients without any apparent structural abnormalities of the urinary tract. These infections may be due to increased pathogenicity of the particular bacteria involved in the infection or may be due to increased susceptibility of the host's vaginal and bladder mucosa to bacterial adherence. On the whole, these 'uncomplicated infections' are usually easily treated and, in fact, clear with a short course of the appropriate antibiotic. UTIs associated with structural or anatomic abnormalities of the urinary tract may allow pathogenic bacteria to enter and persist in the urinary tract, thereby promoting a chronic infection (1). Congenital and acquired abnormalities that interfere with the normal storage and flow of urine within the urinary tract create a complicated setting in which infection is more likely to occur (Table 1). These abnormalities of the urinary tract include obstruction, stasis or reflux, foreign bodies within the urinary tract, and infected urinary stones. A less

Table 1 *Simple classification of disorders that may promote complicated UTIs*

I) Anomaly of urinary system causing obstruction, stasis, or reflux
    A) Prostatic hypertrophy
    B) Neurogenic bladder
    C) Strictures
    D) Vesicoureteral reflux
    E) Other congenital anomalies

II) Foreign body in urinary tract
    A) Urinary catheter, stent, nephrostomy tube, etc.
    B) Instrument manipulation (i.e., cystoscope)

III) Infected urinary stones
    A) Struvite calculi
    B) Secondarily infected calculi

IV) Immunologic or biologic disorders allowing bacterial persistence within urinary tract
    A) Chronic bacterial prostatitis
    B) Chronic cystitis
    C) Immunosuppression
    D) Diabetes
    E) (?Increased susceptibility to pathogen adherence)
    F) (?Chronic pyelonephritis)

---

well-defined group of patients may have a biologic disorder or disease that allows bacterial persistence within the urinary tract.

When the physician suspects a complicated urinary tract infection, aggressive investigation is required to identify the cause and the organism. The initial objective of therapy should be to eliminate the infecting organism and make the patient more comfortable. The definitive management of such patients may involve long-term antibiotic maintenance therapy, surgery or, as is usually the case, both. The optimum treatment should be based on a sound understanding of the pathogenic mechanisms that may be operative in each specific complicated UTI. In the following examples, difficult-to-treat patients are illustrated, and management plans are suggested.

GROUP 1: RECURRENT UTI IN CHILDREN

Case report

A three-year-old girl showed vesicoureteral (VU) reflux on voiding cystourethrogram (VCU) after a documented *Escherichia coli* UTI. She was administered trimethoprim-sulfamethoxazole (TMP-SMX) as low-dose, long-term therapy. However, she developed an allergic skin reaction, and this medication was discontinued. Nitrofurantoin macrocrystals (Macrodantin®) low-dose therapy was instituted, and she was kept on this medication for two years (with appropriate follow-up). A radioisotope VCU showed improvement in the reflux (grade 2). Antibiotics were discontinued by her family physician; however, she developed two documented UTIs over the next two months. Nitrofurantoin macrocrystals therapy was reinstituted and continued for three more years. Radioisoptope VCU done five years after the institution of therapy showed no reflux. The patient has been off antibiotics for 24 months with no UTIs.

Comment

The management of UTI in children is complicated by many factors. The most important factor is the higher incidence in children (compared with adults) of congenital abnormalities predisposing to UTI. Other factors complicating management are 1) the propensity of upper UTI to lead to renal scarring, 2) the associated risk of VU reflux, and 3) concerns regarding chemotherapeutic options and doses for children's infections. The pathogenesis of UTI in children, except for male neonates, is generally assumed to be the same as in adults, involving an ascending infection usually caused by *E. coli* emanating from the bowel flora. Interactions between host factors and bacterial virulence factors are responsible for the establishment of bacteria in the urinary tract. Most UTIs in young children occur in girls. Those girls prone to recurrent infections appear to have periurethral colonization by enteric gram-negative rods; this colonization precedes the ascendance of infection into the bladder and upper urinary tract. Bacterial adhesion to the bladder mucosal surface is the first step in the establishment of infections. In contrast, colonization of bladder urine without adherence or invasion of the bladder mucosa (as occurs in asymptomatic bacteriuria) may be related to a lack of bacterial virulence factors (1–3).

UTIs in children must be approached aggressively. Young children with pyelonephritis are at risk for renal scarring, which can cause hypertension or even chronic renal failure later in life. Renal scarring is associated with VU reflux, particularly when infection and intrarenal reflux are also present. Prompt therapy or prevention of infection is conceivably the most efficient way to prevent renal damage in these children. In most cases, however, some renal scarring is likely to occur and is present at the time of the initial diagnosis.

In all young children the urinary tract must be evaluated after the first UTI. While the intravenous pyelogram is still the classic radiologic investigation, renal ultrasonography is now increasingly used for primary screening of the renal parenchyma and for ruling out dilation of the collecting system. Voiding cystourethrogram to rule out VU reflux, as well as visualization of the urethra in the male, is also included in an adequate screening examination. An isotope VCU might be considered in females, whereas evaluation of the urethral configuration adds nothing to the investigation. Cystoscopy is no longer required as a diagnostic tool in the evaluation of most children with UTIs.

Management of infections in children consists of initial antibiotic treatment based on *in vitro* antibiotic sensitivities. Nitrofurantoin macrocrystals, nitrofurantoin oral suspension, TMP-SMX, nalidixic acid, or amoxicillin may be used for uncomplicated lower UTI. In young children with febrile UTI, prompt therapy is required to abort the inflammatory renal response and, perhaps, decrease the likelihood or extent of renal scarring. Oral medication with TMP-SMX or cephalosporin can be initiated in children who are not septic. The child whose condition is toxic is a candidate for immediate parenteral therapy, possibly with combination therapies such as an aminoglycoside and synthetic penicillin. When the culture and sensitivity results become available, therapy should be switched to a more specific narrow spectrum antibiotic. Long-term, continuous, suppressive therapy should be considered in children with VU reflux and in those with frequent recurrences. Nitrofurantoin macrocrystals and TMP-SMX have proved effective for suppressive therapy in these cases. Those patients with massive VU reflux, breakthrough infections, or failure of the reflux to resolve, may be considered for surgical therapy. Young patients found to have significant congenital abnormalities predisposing them to infections, such as obstruction or stasis, should receive early surgical intervention.

In adults, anomalies of the urinary system causing obstruction or stasis, such as prostatic hypertrophy, neurogenic bladder, or strictures require a slightly different management plan. Prolonged, suppressive antibiotic therapy may be instituted until medical or surgical correction of the anomaly can be achieved. However, in some cases complete normality of the urinary tract cannot be achieved, and prolonged, suppressive antibiotic therapy may be considered.

GROUP 2: CATHETER-ASSOCIATED NOSOCOMIAL INFECTIONS

Case report 1

A 76-year-old man was catheterized because of acute urinary retention. For the next 13 months he was chronically catheterized with Foley catheters in a nursing home. Over that period, he was treated with multiple regimens of antibiotics, including parenteral drugs, for multiple positive cultures. During this time the patient did not have a symptomatic UTI. His last catheter specimens of urine grew multiple organisms resistant to all oral and most parenteral antibiotics. He was admitted to a Queen's University-affiliated hospital with a blocked Foley catheter and sepsis. The catheter was changed and the patient was treated with aggressive antibiotic therapy (netilmicin and ampicillin). Despite therapy he died of overwhelming sepsis. Urine and blood cultures at the time of his emergency admission grew *Serratia marcescens*.

Case report 2

A 44-year-old man with multiple sclerosis had been treated for incontinence with an indwelling catheter for the previous three months. He was admitted to a Queen's University-affiliated hospital with a clinically symptomatic UTI with bladder spasms and fever. The patient's catheter was removed and, after appropriate cultures, he was administered parenteral antibiotics (netilmicin) and intermittent catheterization. Cultures grew *E. coli*. Five days after admission he was discharged home on intermittent catheterization. At home he continued successfully with intermittent catheterization and complained of no further incontinence. However, over the next six weeks he developed two symptomatic UTIs. He began a regimen of low-dose, long-term nitrofurantoin macrocrystals. At six months of follow-up he has continued on intermittent catheterization with no evidence of recurrent UTI.

Comment

The urinary catheter has become an essential part of modern medical care. It is widely used to relieve temporary anatomic or physiologic urinary obstruction, facilitate surgical repair of the urethra and surrounding structures, provide a dry environment for comatose or incontinent patients, and permit accurate measurement of urine output for severely ill patients. Unfortunately, the indwelling catheter presents a hazard to the very patients it is designed to protect and is associated with a significant excess morbidity, high cost, and nearly a threefold increase in mortality among hospitalized patients (4,5).

Infections associated with catheterization are usually mixed. *E. coli* is common, but so are other gram-negative bacilli that are rare in primary infection, such as

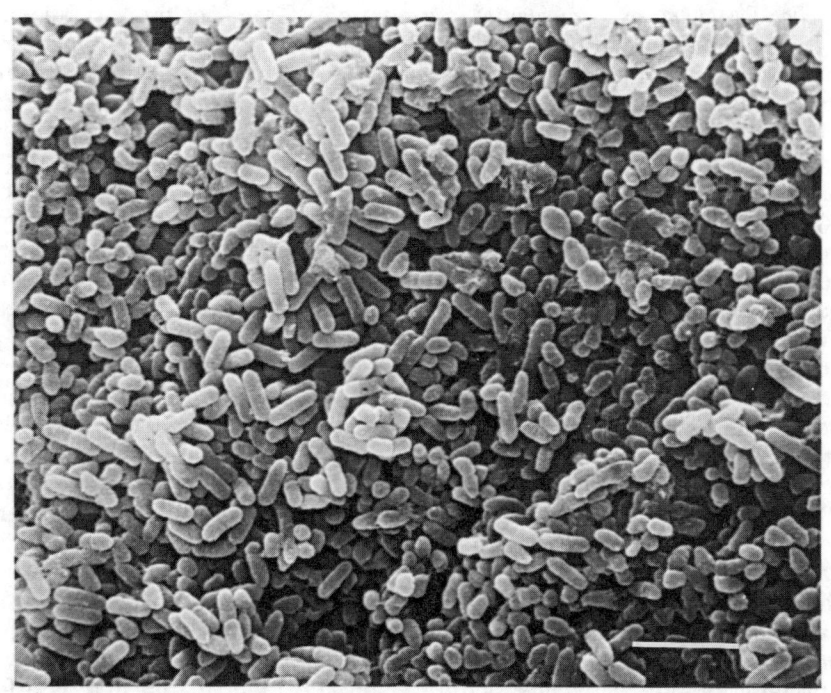

Figure 1a *This specially prepared scanning electron micrograph (SEM) of the surface of a Foley catheter removed from a patient with a* Pseudomonas aeruginosa *UTI clearly depicts the thick bacterial biofilm associated with the catheter. Bar = 5 μm.*

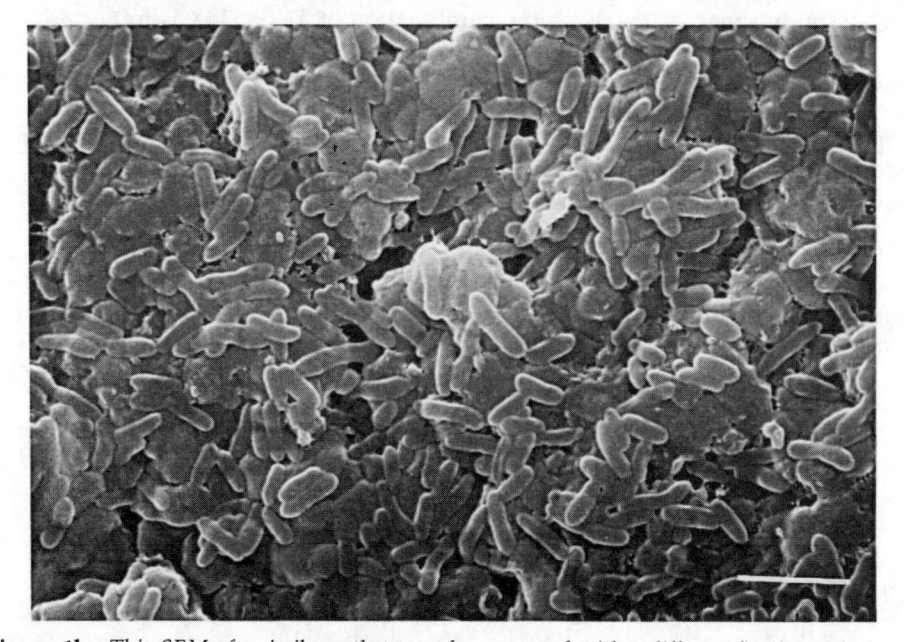

Figure 1b *This SEM of a similar catheter surface prepared with a different fixation technique, demonstrates the bacterial biofilm is incorporated in a slime or glycocalyx matrix. The movement of the glycocalyx-enclosed biofilm up the catheter surfaces appears to be of critical importance in the establishment of a catheter-associated infection. Bar = 5 μm.*

Klebsiella, Pseudomonas, Providentia, Serratia, etc. Gram-positive organisms are also found, including *Streptococcus* and *Staphylococcus*. Bacteria gain entrance to the bladder via a number of mechanisms. Large numbers may be introduced when a catheter is passed, especially if proper aseptic technique is not used. The bacteria may also enter afterward, either through the lumen of the catheter or alongside an indwelling catheter in the periurethral space. These infections are associated with a microscopic bacterial biofilm, which can be many bacteria thick, coating the catheter (6,7) (Figs. 1a,b). The development of the infection appears to involve the intraluminal migration of this bacterial biofilm from an infected drainage spout or, alternatively, ascension of the biofilm along the surface of the catheter in the periurethral space from the urethral meatus (8). Disconnection of the catheter drainage junction will accelerate this process.

Introduction of the closed urinary drainage system has been the most important technologic advance in the development of urinary drainage systems (9). Although these systems have been modified many times over the past two decades, it is not entirely clear whether any of these modifications have appreciably reduced the infection rate. Infections in patients with indwelling catheters occur at a rate of 5% to 10% per day of catheterization, and, at 30 days, almost 100% of catheterized patients will demonstrate bacteriuria (10). In most cases, bacteriuria alone is not remarkable since organisms will appear in the urine without clinical symptoms. Antibiotic therapy in these cases will not eliminate the bacteriuria indefinitely since the antibiotic cannot penetrate the thick bacterial biofilm colonizing the urinary catheter system (11). Antibiotics also select for more resistant organisms within the bacterial biofilm. However, symptomatic infection, manifested as a fever, indicates the organisms are no longer colonizing the urinary tract but have, in fact, invaded the uroepithelium (12). In such cases, the catheter should be removed, or at least changed, and the patient given antibiotics. In less symptomatic patients nitrofurantoin macrocrystals or the combination of TMP-SMX is indicated. For *Pseudomonas* or *Serratia* infections, the treatment of choice is indanyl carbenicillin, tetracycline, or third-generation quinolones (e.g., norfloxacin). Patients who become bacteremic should be treated with parenteral antibiotics. Ampicillin is appropriate for Group D *Streptococcus* and either aminoglycoside or a third-generation cephalosporin would be selected for gram-negative rods. Although antibiotics should be avoided in patients with long-term indwelling Foley catheters, an exception may be made when the organism is *Proteus*. In these patients, encrustation of the catheter and the development of UTI stones become important. Also, patients on intermittent catheterization who develop recurrent infections benefit from low-dose, long-term antibiotic therapy such as nitrofurantoin macrocrystals. Early surgical intervention to keep the period of catheterization as short as possible is perhaps the best method to prevent catheter-associated UTIs. In general, once an indwelling Foley catheter has been introduced, the only accepted methods of reducing the risk of infection are to maintain uninterrupted closed drainage with high standards of nursing care, and to keep the period of catheterization as short as possible (13).

GROUP 3: STRUVITE CALCULI

Case report

A 62-year-old man with a history of chronic *Proteus* UTI that did not clear with appropriate antibiotic therapy had acute systemic sepsis. Intravenous pyelography

(IVP) and tomography clearly demonstrated a large staghorn calculus in the left kidney. A percutaneous nephrostomy was established and the patient was treated with tobramycin. Antibiotic therapy with amoxicillin was instituted after five days of aminoglycoside therapy. Percutaneous ultrasonic debulking of the stone was accomplished followed by extracorporeal shockwave lithotripsy. Four months later, the patient had a *Proteus* UTI, and further investigation revealed a radiolucent stone within the renal pelvis. This recurrent stone was treated with percutaneous ultrasonic lithotripsy followed by one week of renal pelvic irrigation with hemiacidrin. The patient then received low-dose, long-term antibiotic therapy with amoxicillin for two months following discharge. No UTI or recurrent stones were documented during the next 12-month follow-up.

Comment

These struvite and carbonate apatite calculi that occur in the urinary tract are referred to as infection stones because they are always associated with UTIs involving urease-producing bacteria (14). Growth of these stones in the renal pelvis, and extending into the renal calyces, gives them a characteristic staghorn morphology. Extracorporeal shockwave lithotripsy (ESWL) has proved very effective in fragmentation of these stones, either as a monotherapy or after previous debulking by percutaneous ultrasonic lithotripsy (15). Widespread use of antimicrobial agents has markedly reduced the morbidity and mortality associated with the surgical therapies, and urease-inhibitors have shown some early promise.

Urease-producing bacteria, which may originate in the gastrointestinal tract, ascend the urinary tract and colonize uroepithelial cells, forming microcolonies on the epithelial surface enclosed in glycocalyx (bacterial matrix). Urease production by the infecting microorganisms elevates urine pH, at least within the microenvironment of the bacterial colonies, resulting in local precipitation of struvite and apatite crystals in the urine and in the gellike matrix of the bacterial microcolonies (16). The crystals formed within the urine are easily passed and eliminated with voiding; however, those formed within the gellike matrix of the bacterial biofilm are trapped and form the stone nidus within the renal pelvis that subsequently acts as a template for further stone formation (17). These encrusted bacterial microcolonies develop into mature calculi through continued bacterial growth, glycocalyx production and urease activity, crystal deposition, and further incorporation of mucoproteins and mucopolysaccharides (18). The matrix produced both by host material and bacterial matrix protects the uropathogens from host defense mechanisms and antibiotics.

In patients with struvite calculi, appropriate midstream urine collection is required for culture and sensitivity before any stone manipulation. Thorough radiologic investigation of the entire urinary tract is required. In addition to routine IVP, plain film tomograms may be required since the struvite stones can be relatively radiolucent and may be too soft to observe on routine x-ray films. Small fragments left after percutaneous debulking or ESWL are even more difficult to detect. Successful management represents a major urologic challenge and can incorporate open and percutaneous surgery, ESWL, and antibiotic therapy.

The goal of urologic intervention should be entire removal of all fragments of the struvite calculi from the kidney. A less committed approach will usually result in persistence of infection and recurrence of the stone. Although ESWL has been used as a successful monotherapy for struvite staghorn calculi, it is generally accepted that before removing a particularly large struvite staghorn calculus, a percutaneous procedure should be performed to debulk the stone. In some cases the entire stone can be removed via the percutaneous route. In most cases, however, ESWL treatment is employed for the remaining calyceal stone fragments.

Following these combined procedures, a nephrostomy tube can be left in place and percutaneous irrigation with hemiacidrin or other urologic solution may be used in an attempt to dissolve small remaining fragments. Urease inhibitors have been used successfully for treatment of these stones; however, they appear to be more effective in preventing new stone formation or further growth of existing stones than eradicating preexisting stone disease. Urease inhibitors also have very serious side effects that have dampened enthusiasm for their use (19). Antimicrobial therapy should begin at least one week before surgery. A sterile urine culture prior to surgery is ideal. Low-dose, long-term therapy with intravenous antibiotics is essential during the postoperative period. Traditionally the 'penicillin family' of drugs has proved effective in the treatment and prevention of these infection stones. Urine cultures and radiographic follow-up should continue at periodic intervals following stone removal.

GROUP 4: CHRONIC BACTERIAL PROSTATITIS

Case report

A 33-year-old man with a history of undocumented UTI had a three-month history of perineal discomfort, dysuria, frequency, and painful ejaculation for which he had received 10-day courses of tetracycline and ampicillin, respectively. He was referred because of presumed resistance to therapy. At the time of presentation he had not taken any antibiotics for the previous four weeks. A diagnosis of chronic prostatitis was made on physical examination, which disclosed a tender, boggy prostate gland, and on simultaneous quantitative culture, which showed significant counts of *E. coli* in the expressed prostatic secretion. The patient was treated with a three-month course of trimethoprim. At six months' follow-up he had developed no recurrence of symptoms.

Comment

Bacterial infections of the prostate are the most common causes of relapsing recurrent UTIs in men (20). The pathogens responsible for bacterial prostatitis are similar in type and prevalence to those that cause uncomplicated UTIs. Strains of *E. coli* clearly predominate, although other gram-negative rods are found on appropriate cultures. Gram-positive bacteria may also be causative agents in chronic prostatitis. The specific cause of most cases of chronic prostatitis is unknown; however, it is probable that intraprostatic reflux of infected urine serves as the most important mode of prostatic infection (21). There may also be some biologic defect within the prostates of men susceptible to chronic infection; some investigators believe a decreased zinc content in the prostatic fluid may play a role in the pathogenesis of UTI (22). Patients with chronic bacterial prostatitis experience varying degrees of symptomatology, from mild, irritative voiding dysfunction to significant discomfort involving various sites in the lower pelvis and perineum. The prostate is usually tender and somewhat boggy; however, it may also feel quite normal or even indurated. Definitive diagnosis is obtained only with simultaneous quantitative bacteriologic cultures to localize the causative organism in the prostate (23).

Patients with chronic bacterial prostatitis are difficult to cure because of poor diffusion of antimicrobial agents from the plasma into the prostatic secretory system where the bacteria reside (24). A bacterial defense mechanism may also be important. An extensive exopolysaccharide capsule may be produced by bacterial microcolonies in the prostatic ducts (25). Bacteria have evolved this mode of defense in threatened environments, and such encapsulation has been described in other difficult-to-clear human cryptic infections (26). Bacteria may also reside on the surface and within the interstices of prostatic calculi in some patients with this disease; these bacteria would remain difficult to eradicate.

The pharmacologic characteristics of trimethoprim allow for good diffusion into the prostate gland, so this has been a favored therapy for prostatitis. Penicillins, cephalosporins, and nalidixic acid appear to be excluded from the prostatic fluid. Carbenicillin and the new fluoroquinolones (e.g., norfloxacin) have demonstrated efficacy in curing culture-proven chronic prostatitis. Doxycycline and minocycline may possibly be effective in this disease. Therapy should be for six weeks and perhaps longer. Even with appropriate antibiotic therapy over a prolonged time, the cure rate has varied from only 32% to 71% (21–24). In addition to problems with variable cure rates in patients where a bacteriologic diagnosis can be made, confusion arises because of difficulties in obtaining the required specimens, unusual presentations, and difficulties in the diagnosis of other prostatitislike syndromes (i.e., abacterial prostatitis). In those patients whose relapsing UTI is a consequence of persistent prostatitis, the clinician may have to resort to a chronic low-dose, long-term therapy to prevent relapsing UTI. Nitrofurantoin macrocrystals may be an appropriate drug of choice.

DISCUSSION

The approach to treating complicated infections differs significantly from the approach to simple UTI. Therefore, it is important to recognize which situation we are dealing with. Complicated UTIs must be suspected in patients with unusual symptoms or presentation, unusual organisms, failure to clear infection, frequent relapses, or a foreign body. The physician should suspect a complicated infection with any UTI in children. These infections may have minor symptoms or be life-threatening emergencies. They can evolve into serious systemic infections. In any case where a complicated UTI is diagnosed, a diligent search must be made for the cause, as well as for the specific organism.

The clinical examples illustrated in this paper suggest that a clinician can formulate a sound treatment plan if he has an understanding of the pathogenic mechanisms involved in these complicated settings. The appropriate culture and sensitivity-directed antibiotic should be employed for an optimum time.

In uncomplicated UTIs, it is generally accepted that short-term therapy with inexpensive 'front line' antibiotic drugs is adequate, particularly in women. However, in complicated UTIs there is a necessity for broad-spectrum treatment for longer periods of time. The choice of either an oral or a parenteral antibiotic should be dictated by the seriousness of the infection. In most complicated situations, it is important to employ broad spectrum antibiotics that maintain high urine levels but also high drug concentrations in the blood and tissues to ensure eradication of the specific urinary infection, tissue invasion by the bacteria, and possible bacteremia. In seriously ill patients where there is difficulty in presuming the specific pathogen and antibiotic sensitivities, it is essential that drugs that cover the whole range of gram-negative bacteria as well as gram-positive staphylococci and enterococci are used. If possible, single-agent, broad-spectrum antibiotics are preferred over multiple drug combinations. This empiric therapy should be discontinued when specific culture and sensitivity data are available and subsequently changed to more specific narrow-spectrum, possibly oral, therapy.

At the appropriate time urologic or surgical intervention should be employed. This intervention may involve early intubed drainage of the urinary tract, employing either a transurethral or percutaneous approach, or may require a later major surgical procedure or reconstruction. All patients with complicated UTIs should have long-term follow-up and management including surveillance cultures. In many cases there is a need for low-dose, long-term antibiotic therapy. If prolonged therapy is required, the antibiotic should be culture- and disease-specific, have a safe adverse drug-reaction profile, and not cause significant bacterial resistance problems.

REFERENCES

(1) Kunin CM, ed. *Detection, prevention and management of urinary tract infections.* Philadelphia: Lea & Febiger, 1987.
(2) Stamey TA. *Pathogenesis and treatment of urinary tract infection.* Baltimore: Williams & Wilkins Co., 1980.
(3) Winberg J. Urinary tract infections in infants and children. In: Walsh P, Gittes R, Perlmutter A, Stamey TA, eds. *Campbell's urology.* Philadelphia: WB Saunders, 1986: 831–867.
(4) Givens CD, Wenzel RP. Catheter-associated urinary tract infection in surgical patients: a controlled study of the excess morbidity and costs. *J Urol* 1980; **124**: 646–648.
(5) Platt R, Polk BF, Murdock B, Rosner B. Mortality associated with nosocomial urinary tract infection. *N Engl J Med* 1982; **307**: 637–642.
(6) Nickel JC, Gristina AG, Costerton JW. A scanning and transmission electron microscopic study of an infected Foley catheter. *Can J Surg* 1985; **28**: 50–51, 54.
(7) Nickel JC, Downey J, Costerton JW. An ultrastructural study of the microbiological colonization of urinary catheters. *Urology* (in press) 1989.
(8) Nickel JC, Grant SK, Costerton JW. Catheter-associated bacteriuria. An experimental study. *Urology* 1985; **26**: 369–375.
(9) Kunin CM, McCormack RC. Prevention of catheter-induced urinary tract infections by sterile closed drainage. *N Engl J Med* 1966; **274**: 1155–1161.
(10) Warren JW, Muncie HL Jr, Bergquist EJ, Hoopes JM. Sequelae and management of urinary infection in the patient requiring chronic catheterization. *J Urol* 1981; **125**: 1–8.
(11) Nickel JC, Ruseska I, Wright JB, Costerton JW. Tobramycin resistance of *Pseudomonas aeruginosa* cells growing as a biofilm on urinary catheter material. *Antimicrob Agents Chemother* 1985; **27**: 619–624.
(12) Daifuku R, Stamm WE. Bacterial adherence to bladder uroepithelial cells in catheter-associated urinary tract infection. *N Engl J Med* 1986; **314**: 1208–1213.
(13) Stamm WE. Guidelines for prevention of catheter-associated urinary tract infection. *Ann Intern Med* 1975; **82**: 386–390.
(14) Griffith DP. Struvite stones. *Kidney Int* 1978; **13**: 372–382.
(15) Wilson JWL, Nickel JC, Nolan R. Percutaneous renal surgery. *Can J Surg* 1987; **30**: 389–391.
(16) McLean RJC, Nickel JC, Noakes VC, Costerton JW. An *in vitro* ultrastructural study of infectious kidney stone genesis. *Infect Immun* 1985; **49**: 805–811.
(17) Nickel JC, Olson M, McLean RJC, Grant SK, Costerton JW. An ecological study of infected urinary stone genesis in an animal model. *Br J Urol* 1987; **59**: 21–30.
(18) Nickel JC, Emtage J, Costerton JW. Ultrastructural microbial ecology of infection-induced urinary stones. *J Urol* 1985; **133**: 622–627.

(19) Bagley DH. Pharmacologic treatment of infection stones. *Urol Clin North Am* 1987; **14**: 347-352.
(20) Meares EM Jr. Prostatitis: a review. *Urol Clin North Am* 1975; **2**: 3-27.
(21) Meares EM Jr. Etiology of prostatitis. *Urology* 1984; **24** (suppl): 4-5.
(22) Fair WR, Couch J, Wehner N. Prostatic antibacterial factor: identity and significance. *Urology* 1976; **7**: 169-177.
(23) Meares EM, Stamey TA. Bacteriologic localization patterns in bacterial prostatitis and urethritis. *Invest Urol* 1968; **5**: 492-518.
(24) Sharer WC, Fair WR. The pharmacokinetics of antimicrobic diffusion in chronic bacterial prostatitis. *Prostate* 1982; **3**: 139-148.
(25) Nickel JC, Olson M, Costerton JW. Pathogenesis of chronic bacterial prostatitis (submitted for publication).
(26) Costerton JW, Cheng KJ, Geesey GG, *et al*. Bacterial biofilms in nature and disease. *Annu Rev Microbiol* 1987; **41**: 435-464.

Women's attitudes and the treatment of urinary tract infections

M. Elhilali

Department of Urology, Royal Victoria Hospital and McGill University, Montreal, Quebec, Canada

ABSTRACT

Women's concerns about urinary tract infections (UTIs) include physical discomfort, expense of medication, and information regarding reinfection. In 1987, a telephone survey was conducted regarding women's attitudes and beliefs about UTIs and the treatment received from physicians from UTIs. By random selection of 819 households, researchers identified 201 women between the ages of 14 and 65 years who had previously sought medical treatment for a UTI. These women were questioned on symptoms, occurrence rates, causes, and treatment of UTIs. Over 90% of them rated the care they received from physicians as good or excellent. Reasons for dissatisfaction ranged from recurrence of the problem to lack of explanation from the physician. Respondents showed a strong interest in learning more about the cause and treatment of UTIs from their physicians. Reinfections can frequently be treated successfully with the original, first-line antibiotic, thereby not alienating the patient by selection of more expensive medication. Successful treatment of UTIs should address patient concerns as well as the infection.

INTRODUCTION

It is appropriate for us to include in our Consensus on Management of Urinary Tract Infection a discussion of the interaction of physician and patient. Lower urinary tract infection (LUTI) is one of the most common problems seen in medical practice. Women are especially susceptible; an estimated 20% of all women experience symptoms of urinary tract infection (UTI) at some point during their lifetime (1). Although physicians regard UTI as an ordinary problem, most patients do not find it ordinary at all. The discomfort of a first-time UTI can be alarming to a young woman, and recurrent or chronic UTI may be both annoying and worrisome, especially if a relationship to sexual activity is perceived. In addition, repeated office visits and prescription costs can create considerable burdens.

The patient's anxiety together with our earnest desire to get rid of this bothersome type of case may tempt us to attack the problem with unnecessary vigor. This temptation should be resisted; for the simple infection, a simple treatment approach is most suited. Each of us should develop a private formulary of drugs with which we are familiar and comfortable. Just as the infectious disease specialist in the hospital maintains a clear distinction between first-line antibiotics and reserve drugs, in our own practices, each of us should draw a line between those drugs which we regularly use for routine cases and those we reserve for more serious infections. This strategy allows us to deal effectively with resistant organisms and serious infections when they occur.

Proper diagnosis is another critical part of effective therapy. It is important to differentiate between UTI and other conditions that can mimic it. Careful questioning of the patient can provide valuable clues to diagnosis, such as whether the onset of symptoms was abrupt—which would point to UTI—or gradual, which suggest vaginitis or sexually transmitted disease (STD) (2). Ascertaining what is typical for a particular patient will help the clinician determine a disease (2).

Furthermore, successful therapy should address the patient's concerns as well as her infection. It is our obligation to provide education and reassurance along with each prescription.

First, let's consider a common scenario. A young woman has recurrent or persistent symptoms, and her urine is sterile. Diagnosis is usually by exclusion. We call it 'urethral syndrome', but we are ignorant of the underlying cause. An antibiotic is prescribed, providing temporary respite. When medication is stopped, the symptoms recur. The patient expresses dissatisfaction, and a different antibiotic is prescribed. With each successive recurrence, against our better judgment, therapy becomes more exotic and more expensive. We may try urethral dilatation or urethrotomy, which may work, but we don't know why. In frustration, some urologists may turn to injecting periurethral steroids or using intraurethral inserts. What drives us to overtreat for this particular syndrome? Perhaps it is the knowledge that we are being rated by the patient.

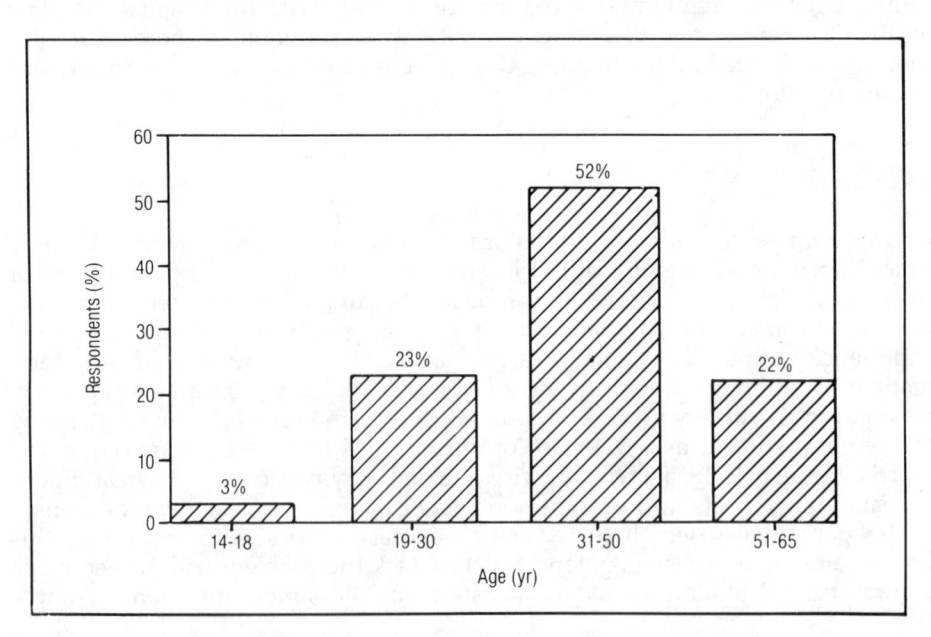

Figure 1 *A telephone survey of 819 households produced 201 respondents from ages 14 to 65 who had experienced some type of urinary tract infection. Fifty-two percent were in the 31 to 50 age-group.*

THE SURVEY

In September 1987, the T. A. Miller Company, a Clifton, New Jersey, health-care marketing research firm, conducted a UTI study via telephone interviews with randomly selected households throughout the United States. Of 4299 telephone calls, the yield was 819 admissible interviews. Out of this sample, the researchers identified 201 female respondents between the ages of 14 and 65 years who had previously had a UTI that caused them to see a doctor for treatment.

Patient age-groups, income, marital status

The demographics of the sample were as follows: 3% of the respondents were 14 to 18 years of age; 23% were 19 to 30; 52% were 31 to 50; and 22% were 51 to 65 (Fig. 1). The average age of the study participants was 39.9 years. Six percent of the women said their first UTI had occurred when they were younger than age 14. Fifteen percent said they had their first UTI between 14 and 18. The overwhelming majority, 60%, reported their first UTI to have occurred between 19 and 30. Thirteen percent reported a first UTI at 31 to 50 years of age and 3% at ages 51 to 65 (Fig. 2). Three percent responded that they did not know or could not recall. The mean age at which UTIs first occurred in this population was 25.9 years. Young women comprise a large proportion of the UTI cases we treat.

The average total annual household income of study participants who supplied this information was $28 510, with a range from under $15 000 to over $50 000. Seventy percent of the respondents were married, 17% were single, and 10% were divorced (Fig. 3). Three percent declined to reveal their marital status. Twenty percent had no children, 15% had one child, 30% had two, and 33% had three or more children (Fig. 4). Two individuals did not answer the question. One woman in five (20%) became sexually active between the ages of 14 and 16, 42% between ages 17 and 19%, and most of the others in their early 20s.

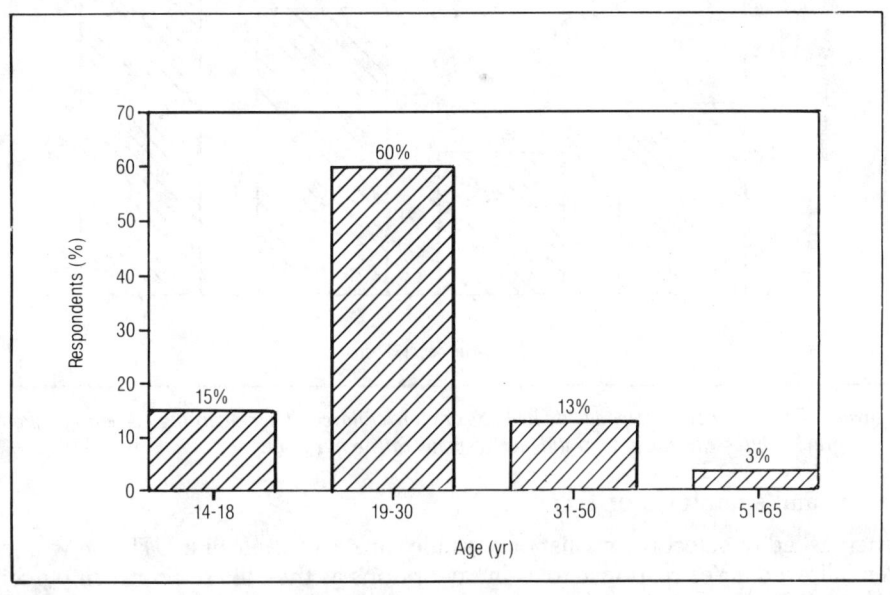

Figure 2 *Of the sample discussed in Fig. 1, the overwhelming majority of first UTIs occurred at ages 19 to 30 (60%), with 21% before age 19 and a smaller percent after age 30.*

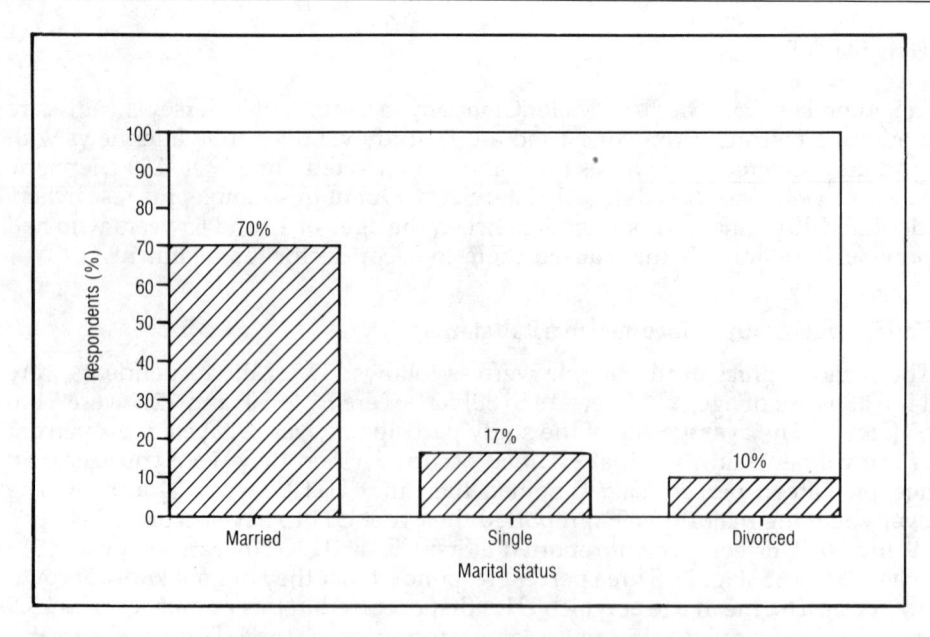

Figure 3 *Seventy percent of the women who had had UTIs were married, 17% were single, 10% divorced, and 3% declined to reveal their marital status.*

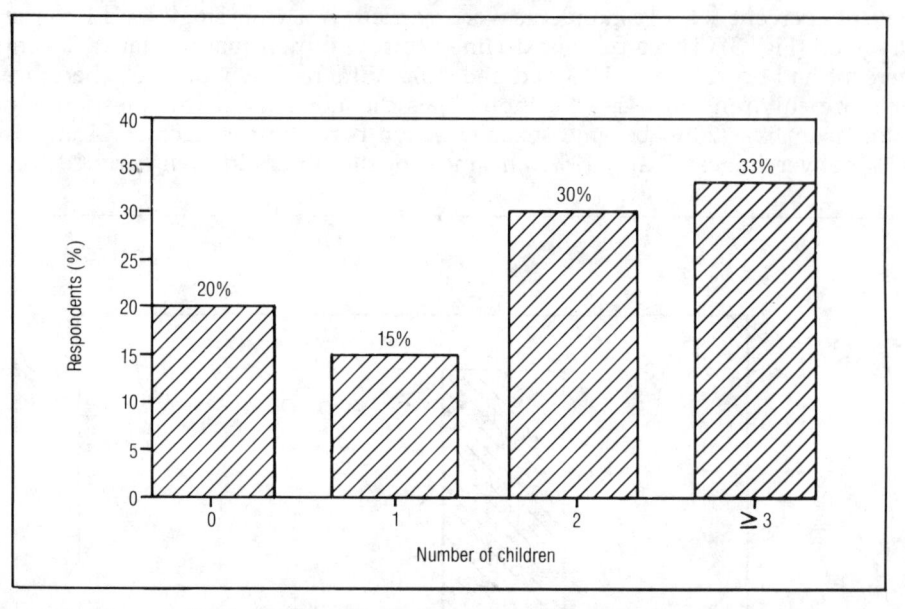

Figure 4 *The majority of respondents had one or more children. The remaining percent not shown in the graph represents those who did not respond to the question.*

Causes and symptoms of UTI

When asked to select from a list of possible causes of their first UTI, the women were allowed a Yes response to as many options as they liked. Fourteen percent blamed tight clothing or pantyhose, and 12% blamed sexual activity (Table 1). Other causes in descending order of selection, included soapy bathwater and

Table 1 Patients' perceptions of UTI causes

	Respondents[a]
Tight clothing or pantyhose	14
Sexual activity	12
Soapy bathwater/bubble baths	11
Too many soft drinks	11
Pregnancy	9
First sexual experience (honeymoon cystitis)	6
Too many sweets	4
Poor personal hygiene	3
Bathing suits	3
Dieting	3
Hot tubs/health clubs	1
Don't know	27

[a] Respondents were allowed to choose more than one answer.

Table 2 Symptoms of UTI

	Respondents[a] (%)
Burning micturition	89
Frequent urination	82
Bladder pain	57
Back pain	52
Fever	19
Nausea	8
Itching	4
Blood in the urine	4

[a] Symptoms were reported by 201 respondents who qualified for inclusion in the study following a 1987 telephone survey of 819 households.

bubble baths (11%), too many soft drinks (11%), pregnancy (9%), first sexual experience—honeymoon cystitis (6%), too many sweets (4%), poor personal hygiene (3%), bathing suits (3%), dieting (3%), and hot tubs and health clubs (1%). Twenty-seven percent of the respondents did not know the possible cause of their UTI . . . and, in many cases, we probably won't be able to pinpoint a cause either. Overall, certain risk factors appear to predispose patients to UTIs. These risk factors include diabetes, immune deficiency, structural abnormalities, and possibly sexual habits.

Major symptoms associated with UTIs in this sample were typical: burning pain when urinating (89%), frequent urination (82%), bladder pain (57%), back pain (52%), fever (19%), nausea (8%), itching (4%), and blood in the urine (4%) (Table 2).

Sexual concerns

Subjects were also asked whether they thought their first UTI was a punishment for having had sex. Of the respondents, 57% said No, and 31% declined to answer; however, 10% of the women indicated this to be true. Two percent did not know. That a woman is more likely to have a UTI if she is sexually active was accepted by 52%; 24% disagreed, 23% were uncertain, and 1% did not answer. However, only 11% of respondents thought women who have UTIs are likely to be viewed as promiscuous or sexually active.

Nearly two women in five (38%) said they have altered their sexual activity because of a UTI. Among them, 77% abstained from sex. An additional 9% said they had 'less sexual activity', and 7% opted to use a birth control method different from the pill, primarily condoms.

Forty percent of the women indicated that a sexual partner can transmit a UTI, while 32% disagreed, and 27% were uncertain. However, only about one woman in six (17%) considered UTI to be an STD. Nevertheless, approximately four out of five respondents (79%) said they were to some degree concerned about STDs, and 92% said the incidence of STDs was increasing somewhat or significantly.

Although most women did not associate UTIs with STDs, 17% assumed that having a UTI would increase their chances of getting an STD, and 13% thought a UTI would increase a woman's risk of contracting acquired immunodeficiency syndrome.

Type of care received

Which medical specialists did women see for a UTI? In this sample in which some women answered to more than one choice, 55% said they saw an obstetrician/gynecologist, 11% saw a urologist, and 48% visited a general practitioner or family practitioner (Table 3).

Overall, the study reflected a 24% incidence in households in the United States, in which a female had previously had a UTI and had been treated by a physician. The study indicates that in approximately one household in four throughout this country, a woman has previously been treated for a UTI. These patients were overwhelmingly positive about the type of care they received from physicians. Forty-nine percent described their care as excellent, 42% as good. However, 18 respondents (9%) rated their care as fair or poor (Table 4). The reasons for dissatisfaction among the 18 patients included recurrence of symptoms and physician-related problems: lack of an explanation, his 'not knowing what he was talking about' or taking too long to figure out what was wrong, implication that the UTI was caused by sexual activity, or disbelief that the patient truly had a UTI. Whereas one patient was dissatisfied because the physician treated the problem but did not prescribe any medication, another complained that medication was prescribed to which she was allergic.

On the positive side, 90% of the women said the physician had answered their questions, and 69% said the reason why UTIs occur had been explained. At the time of their office visits for a urinary tract problem, 99% of the women received

Table 3 *Physicians visited for UTI*

	Respondents (%)
Obstetrician/gynecologist	55
General practitioner/family practitioner	48
Urologist	11

Table 4 *Patients' ratings of physician care*

	Respondents (%)
Excellent	49
Good	42
Fair/poor	9

Table 5 *Patients' sources of information about UTI*

	Respondents (%)
Physicians	92
Women's magazines	52
Family or friends	51
Close friend	50
Television talk show	48
Pharmacists	46

prescriptions for medication and 75% received an explanation of the kind of medication being given and its purpose. Two thirds of the women whose physicians did not explain why the UTI occurred indicated that they had wanted the information. Although the opinions are interesting, the fact that 99% of these women were ready to answer the question 'What type of care did you receive?' was more so. We can conclude from this that we are all being graded by our patients. No wonder we feel under pressure to perform!

Sources of information

By what standard are we being measured? How do women get their information about the right way to treat UTI? It is a relief to find from the survey that 92% turn to physicians for information. However, women's magazines, television, pharmacists, and family or friends are also important sources of information (Table 5). Many patients have garnered information from the above sources or in some other manner developed opinions about the etiology of this disorder.

Recurrence of UTI

Slightly more than one third (34%) of the respondents reported a recurrent UTI after initial treatment. The risk of recurrence increased with patient age, ranging from a 25% level for patients aged 14 to 30, up to a 38% level of recurrence for patients aged 51 to 65 years.

Recurrences were markedly higher among divorced women (52%) as compared with married (33%) or single women (32%). Among women who developed recurrences of UTI, 6% said the recurrence was immediate, 43% said the recurrence developed within six weeks after treatment, and 43% said the recurrence developed beyond six weeks after treatment. Women who had no answer or could not remember accounted for the remaining percentage.

Opinion of UTI treatment

The medical profession has gone through a variety of conventional wisdoms as to the proper way to treat recurrent UTIs. These include long-term therapy, urethral dilatation, internal urethrotomy, periurethral steroids, and intraurethral suppositories (Table 6). To my knowledge, no controlled studies have been done demonstrating any of these treatments to be more effective than simple, first-line antibiotic therapy. In light of this, perhaps we should not be too critical of the patient's views on how best to treat UTIs. Eighty-seven percent replied that they should drink fluids. Other responses included: take antibiotics (79%), reduce sexual activity (27%), stop sexual activity (22%), take aspirin or Tylenol® (16%), eat yogurt and health foods (8%), or drink cranberry juice (5%).

Table 6 Management choices[a]

Antibiotics
More expensive antibiotics
Long-term antibiotics
Urethral dilatation
Internal urethrotomy
Periurethral steroids
Intraurethral suppository

[a] Ranked in ascending order for simple acute to stubborn recurrent infections.

Table 7 Patients' perceptions of medication costs

	Respondents (%)
Inexpensive	43
Expensive	28
Moderate	3
No opinion	24
No answer	2

First-line treatment for uncomplicated UTI should be antibiotics; they are usually effective. However, because of host factors or the organism itself, we sometimes encounter failure or recurrence, eliciting the response 'change antibiotics', which may not always be appropriate. Most recurrent infections are actually new infections and will respond well to the original antibiotic. There may be no reason to administer more expensive therapy. We are all aware that expensive medication alienates a number of patients. In the telephone survey, 28% of patients considered their medication to be expensive (Table 7). If expensive drugs are called for, and we fail to explain the situation thoroughly, the patient will lose patience and confidence.

Patient education

Women want to learn more about UTIs. Even though 90% of those surveyed said the physician had answered their questions, and 69% said the physician had explained why UTIs occur, 42% were interested in learning even more about UTIs. In fact, an overwhelming 92% of these women said they rely on their physician to provide such additional information. This suggests a need for physicians to use patient education materials when treating women who have UTIs.

CONCLUSION

As these data suggest, women are very concerned about UTIs—perhaps more so than any of us realized. In this paper, we have discussed our approaches to treatment. However, we cannot lose sight of our patients' concerns. As physicians, we must provide the information women want, as well as the treatment they need.

REFERENCES

(1) Andriole VT. Urinary tract infections: recent developments. *J Infect Dis* 1987; **156**: 865–869.
(2) Tuomala R. Confronting issues that sidetrack optimal care. *Contemp Obstet Gynecol* 1988; **32**(4): 109.

Managing uncomplicated urinary tract infections: A worldwide consensus

SESSION I

ROUNDTABLE DISCUSSION: **Consensus on selecting therapy for simple UTIs**
C. Lowell Parsons, MD,
Moderator

Dr Parsons: How important is it to determine definitively whether an upper UTI is present?

Dr Harrison: It's not that important. With our antimicrobial agents, treatment can be started in patients with favorable histories and minimal clinical findings. However, single-dose therapy is sometimes suggested as a means of localizing the infection. What is your opinion of this, Dr Harding?

Dr Harding: It's a controversial area. Robert H. Rubin, MD, at Harvard Medical School, and his colleagues conducted a multicenter study comparing single-dose therapy with 10-day therapy in an indigent population. Some patients on single-dose therapy developed subclinical pyelonephritis without upper tract symptoms.

Dr Harrison: Different age-groups and populations may have different responses to single-dose therapy. A poorer, urban population may have a 45% response compared with 80% to 85% in rural areas. Single-dose therapy is in a state of flux. Patients need more than one day of therapy because their symptoms last at least 48 to 72 h.

Dr Harding: From a practical point of view, with persistent symptoms and inflammation, the patient wants longer treatment.

Dr Moseley: Dr Parsons, you presented the scientific criteria for drug choice. What drug do you think is used the most?

Dr Parsons: By my criteria, TMP-SMX is not a logical first-line antibiotic. However, its widespread use leads me to believe it's being considered as such.

Management of urinary tract infections, edited by Lloyd H. Harrison, 1990; Royal Society of Medicine Services International Congress and Symposium Series No. 154, published by Royal Society of Medicine Services Limited.

Dr Moseley: I understand that trimethoprim on its own was never fully evaluated before it was combined with sulfamethoxazole.

Dr Brumfitt: The original studies showed rapid emergence of resistance to trimethoprim alone. I don't think sulfamethoxazole is synergistic in preventing resistance, nor is there an indication for it.

Dr Moseley: In my use of the combination, most of the adverse effects come from the sulfonamide, and many doctors are not aware that in the British National Formulary, TMP-SMX is contraindicated in the elderly.

Dr Parsons: TMP-SMX is more appropriately held in reserve for use when other, simpler antibiotics fail. Many physicians in the United States don't realize that the package insert for TMP-SMX recommends that initial episodes of uncomplicated urinary tract infections be treated with a single, effective antibacterial agent, rather than this combination product.

Dr Harding: Dr Van Cangh, you mentioned a few patients who showed significant resistance to norfloxacin. Were they catheterized and therefore more prone to develop resistant bacteria with any antibiotic?

Dr Van Cangh: Yes, several patients with catheters did develop resistant strains.

Dr Brumfitt: Looking at the number of new quinolones available and the number of indications for which they are promoted, Dr Julian Davis, chairman of microbiology at the Pasteur Institute, estimated that there would be wide resistance to fluoroquinolones in two to two and one-half years. In your survey, norfloxacin was the second most often used drug, after nitrofurantoin macrocrystals. Do you know why this expensive drug was used so often?

Dr Van Cangh: There is no restriction on drug usage in Belgium, and norfloxacin has been widely advertised, especially for uncomplicated cystitis. The broad use of such potent new medications should be controlled in some way.

Dr Parsons: I believe that there are many similarities in the way we think uncomplicated UTIs should be treated, regardless of where we're practicing. Judging from the papers presented, there appears to be consensus that simple UTIs can generally be treated without much laboratory testing or use of invasive procedures. Furthermore, for most of us, single-dose therapy is not the treatment of choice.

We all are concerned that the bacteria common in UTIs will become resistant to many of the antimicrobials available. Older, well-proven antibiotics, such as nitrofurantoin macrocrystals, adequately eliminate infection in most patients with acute UTI. Nitrofurantoin macrocrystals does this perhaps better and certainly more cost-effectively than newer drugs. Moreover, the development of resistance to nitrofurantoin has rarely been reported.

SESSION 2

ROUNDTABLE DISCUSSION: **Consensus on utility of Macrodantin® in UTI**
Ernesto Calderón-Jaimes, MD
Moderator

Dr Bint: Are there any reports of transferable, plasmid-mediated resistance to nitrofurantoin?

Dr McOsker: Although the incorporation of nitrofurantoin resistance into an R factor has been reported, it was not isolated in a clinical setting. The *Escherichia coli* we obtained by mutagenesis is almost certainly a reductase-loss mutant that is not transferable. One thing that may mitigate against that kind of resistance *in vivo* is that reductase activity seems to be distributed fairly evenly over several different systems in the bacterium.

Dr Calderón-Jaimes: Does nitrofurantoin activity require reductive activation or are there circumstances under which unreduced nitrofurantoin could be active?

Dr McOsker: Nitrofurantoin, under some special circumstances, may not require reductive activation to kill bacteria. In the laboratory, under conditions where no reductive activation could be demonstrated, the *E. coli* bacteria were killed, and, in fact, the minimum inhibitory concentration (MIC) remained the same. Therefore, some reductase-negative mutants may be susceptible. This may help to explain the effect of pH on the sensitivity of *Proteus* to nitrofurantoin. Once the pH is sufficiently lowered, nitrofurantoin may be able to enter *Proteus* cells, and it may still be active.

Dr Bint: Does the nonspecific mode of action of nitrofurantoin have any implication for mammalian cells?

Dr McOsker: There seems to be no demonstrable toxic effect on human cells. Toxicity may not be observed because of the pharmacokinetics of nitrofurantoin. The serum half-life of nitrofurantoin is about 19 min, and biodistribution after that is almost exclusively in the urine. It may be that the concentrations in the serum are so low that entry into mammalian cells is never a clinical problem. Toxicity to the bladder epithelium may not occur because the glycocalyx on the epithelial cells prevents entry. The real answer is an empiric, clinical one: Nitrofurantoin has been used for 35 years with no apparent effect on human cells.

Dr Harrison: Dr Brumfitt, if you have a pregnant patient with a history of recurrent UTI, is there a case for low-dose, long-term therapy before she becomes infected, even before she has bacteriuria?

Dr Brumfitt: If she is in her 30s and has been trying to become pregnant for some time, I would continue low-dose, long-term therapy with an appropriate antibacterial agent throughout pregnancy. I think that in this situation the potential benefits of therapy outweigh the risks.

Dr Mulholland: I've been asked by practitioners which drugs are safest, especially during the first trimester of pregnancy. There are really no drugs that don't have some side effects in pregnancy. How would you rank various classes of drugs for safety during pregnancy?

Dr Brumfitt: In the United Kingdom we follow the indications in the National Formulary. Nitrofurantoin and ampicillin are not expressly contraindicated during pregnancy, whereas all the new oral cephalosporins carry pregnancy warnings.

Dr Calderón-Jaimes: Although I think we have arrived at a consensus that nitrofurantoin is usually the best choice for uncomplicated UTIs, the subject matter of this roundtable has had a wider range than was suggested by its title. We have discussed the mechanisms of antibacterial activity and optimal dosing and have concluded with a discussion of treating pregnant patients who have bacteriuria. Dr McOsker has suggested good reasons why clinical resistance to nitrofurantoin macrocrystals hasn't been observed, but there are still some interesting puzzles about its entry into the cell. Also, most of us think that for most patients, 50 to 100 mg qid is the optimum dose for the treatment of acute cases. For low-dose, long-term therapy 50 to 100 mg at bedtime may be adequate. For the patient with recurrent infections, there isn't a clear consensus about the roles of low-dose, long-term therapy, intermittent self-treatment, and postcoital dosing. Certainly, however, patient compliance, education, and motivation are critical to successful treatment. Low-dose, long-term antibiotic therapy during pregnancy appears to be warranted in special cases, such as for older patients with histories of recurrent UTIs.

SESSON 3

ROUNDTABLE DISCUSSION: **Consensus of the management of UTIs**
Mostafa Elhilali, MD,
Moderator

Dr Harding: Dr Van Kerrebroeck, what was the incidence of *Staphylococcus saprophyticus* infection in the study at your hospital?

Dr Van Kerrebroeck: We had 26 patients with staphylococcal infections out of 244 patients from whom we got isolates. Among these 26 patients, 16 had coagulase-negative and 10 had coagulase-positive staphylococcal infections. I don't know how many were *S. saprophyticus*.

Dr Harding: There are, of course, many types of coagulase-negative staphylococci. We found that young, sexually active female outpatients are prone to *S. saprophyticus*.

Dr Brumfitt: Staphylococcal UTIs are important because they can cause pyelonephritis.

Dr Harding: The prevalence of bacteriuria is high in diabetic patients. No one knows why, but decreased chemotactic factors are one theory. How should UTIs in diabetic patients be treated? Should diabetic patients with asymptomatic bacteriuria always be treated? I think they should because these patients tend to receive instrumentation often, and, as a rule of thumb, bacteriuria should be treated before any kind of instrumentation is used. The risk of pyelonephritis is another consideration. Diabetic patients are one of the subgroups in whom renal function can actually deteriorate with acute pyelonephritis.

Dr Brumfitt: If a patient's diabetes is well controlled, bouts of asymptomatic bacteriuria and symptomatic attacks generally are not severe. However, in the presence of uncontrolled diabetes, infections are likely to be serious. Deterioration in leukocyte function has been demonstrated during periods of unstable diabetes, and that may partially explain the etiology. Diabetic patients are also more likely to incur renal infections.

Dr Parsons: Diabetic patients will not necessarily have more frequent bladder infections, unless they have structural abnormalities related to long-term changes. This may be because the immune system plays no role in protecting the bladder from infection. Women who are immunosuppressed after kidney transplantation also show little difference in the frequency of bacteriuria. The keys to bladder defense are mechanical washing and emptying, combined with surface glycoproteins that prevent bacterial adherence. However, renal lesions are more frequent in diabetic patients who have recurrent infections than they are in nondiabetic patients.

Dr Brumfitt: Diabetic patients are also more likely to incur renal infections.

Dr Parsons: Yes. The bacteria are different in renal and bladder infections. The mechanism of renal infection in the normal individual is probably hematogenous spread, making the differences in immune function of the two organs more significant.

Dr Harding: Dr Mulholland, we have compared self-treatment and continuous and intermittent low-dose, long-term therapy and found that patients preferred continuous low-dose, long-term therapy because they didn't have to dread the next infection. What do you find?

Dr Mulholland: It doesn't make sense to withdraw treatment from patients if those patients have had continuous low-dose, long-term therapy for a year after a very difficult time previously with multiple infections. However, if such patients can stop taking medication and stay well for three or four months, that is good.

I've been surprised that self-medication has received so much criticism because I like it, and it has helped me in my practice. Of course, patients must be educated, but we keep careful records of each treatment episode, and patients keep annual appointments.

Dr Parsons: Patients may have cycles of infections, and perhaps low-dose, long-term therapy breaks the cycles, allowing the bladder epithelium to recover over two to three months. The bladders of patients with recurrent UTIs may not be normal for many weeks.

Dr Elhilali: Dr Nickel, how do you select patients for low-dose, long-term therapy?

Dr Nickel: Patients with neurogenic bladders and intermittent catheterization do very well on low-dose long-term nitrofurantoin macrocrystals. Another group of patients who do well on long-term antibiotic therapy are those waiting for surgery. Long-term suppressive therapy should be considered for those patients with long-term bacterial persistence secondary to an infection focus within the prostate.

Dr Harding: Are immunocompromised patients candidates for low-dose, long-term therapy?

Dr Nickel: They can be, even though there are risks. It is a good idea to take a stent out or change to a new one under antibiotic coverage.

Dr Elhilali: Although we have discussed a number of issues in this session, including low-dose, long-term therapy and infections in diabetics, I think, in all three sessions, the key point is in our treatment of simple versus complicated infections. Simple infections should be treated by simple means, using first-line agents, such as nitrofurantoin macrocrystals. Treatment should be short and pulsed at each episode. In contrast, complicated infections require multiple, diverse approaches.

Dr Harrison: I've found that there is a kind of international consensus: As urologists, we're doing fewer invasive procedures such as cystoscopies and urethral dilatation. Because 90% of UTIs are uncomplicated, we're relying more on antibiotics. However, the profusion of new antimicrobials has needlessly complicated the clinical picture and made treatment rather expensive for these patients. But we've heard today that we can still expect excellent cost-effective results with proven agents in uncomplicated UTIs.

Uncomplicated Urinary Tract Infections: Determining Appropriate Therapy

CME TEST

Please use the answer card below to record your answers to the following questions.

This program will qualify for 3 hours Category 1 CME credit until February, 1992. After that date, tests will be corrected, but CME credit will not be awarded. A minimum passing grade of 78% (18 of 23 answers correct) is necessary to qualify for CME credit.

A corrected answer sheet will be returned to you with a record of the credits you have earned.

Harrison

1. The most clinically reliable test for distinguishing simple from complicated UTI and determining the site of infection is:
   (a) A leukocyte count
   (b) Bilateral ureteral catheterization
   (c) Bladder washout
   (d) Antibody-coated-bacteria tests

2. Women with recurrent UTIs, despite anatomically normal tracts, usually have:
   (a) Stones
   (b) Foreign bodies
   (c) Obstructions
   (d) Increased bacterial adherence to vaginal epithelium

Parsons

3. All but one of the following are criteria guiding the selection of a urinary tract antibiotic:
   (a) The agent should have a minimal effect on normal intestinal and vaginal flora
   (b) The drug selected should cover both aerobic and anaerobic flora
   (c) The antibiotic must attain adequate urinary concentrations
   (d) Total cost should be low

4. Urinary tract specificity of an antibiotic is a desirable characteristic for all but one of the following reasons:
   (a) Altered intestinal flora become a reservoir for subsequent urinary tract infections
   (b) Disruption of vaginal flora can promote yeast overgrowth and vaginitis
   (c) Resistance to agents with broad tissue distribution may render them ineffective in other non-urinary-tract infections
   (d) Serum levels of agents with broader distribution must be monitored

Van Cangh

5. What percentage of all women experience at least one episode of acute lower UTI in their lifetimes?
   (a) 50%
   (b) 80%
   (c) 20%
   (d) 10%

Gomez

6. Nitrofurantoin macrocrystals was shown to be significantly better *in vitro* than TMP/SMX for all but one of the following reasons:
   (a) A large number of gram-positive and gram-negative strains were found susceptible to nitrofurantoin macrocrystals
   (b) 94% of bacterial strains of patients completing the study were susceptible to nitrofurantoin macrocrystals, compared with 77% susceptible to TMP/SMX
   (c) Only *Klebsiella oxytoca* were resistant to nitrofurantoin macrocrystals
   (d) All of the *E. coli* strains were susceptible to nitrofurantoin macrocrystals

7. Although the overall success rates for nitro-furantoin macrocrystals and TMP/SMX were equivalent, the former agent may be preferable because:
   (a) Women have more urinary tract infections, and prefer nitrofurantoin
   (b) There were more side effects with TMP/SMX
   (c) The TMP/SMX cure rate may be "inflated", since most of the patients with strains of *E. coli* resistant to TMP/SMX were randomly assigned to treatment with nitrofurantoin macrocrystals.
   (d) It is easier to obtain TMP/SMX without prescription

McOsker

8. A newly described mechanism of action of nitrofurantoin macrocrystals:
   (a) Inhibition of bacterial protein synthesis at the ribosomal level
   (b) Interference with bacterial cell wall synthesis
   (c) Interference with bacterial DNA synthesis
   (d) Competitive binding with penicillin-binding proteins

The Bowman Gray School of Medicine is accredited by the Accreditation Council for Continuing Medical Education (ACCME) to sponsor continuing medical education for physicians. This program is designated as meeting the criteria for 3 credit hours in Category 1 for the Physician's Recognition Award of the American Medical Association.

9. One of the following statements is false:
   (a) Nitrofurantoin is effective against more than 90% of urinary tract pathogens
   (b) The lack of significant resistance to nitrofurantoin is probably due to the large number of target proteins
   (c) Use of nitrofurantoin macrocrystals can help preserve the long-term efficacy of newer agents, such as the quinolones
   (d) The lack of resistance to nitrofurantoin thirty years after its introduction is probably explained by its infrequent use

Ellis and Moseley
10. Criteria for a lower urinary tract infection include all but one of the following:
    (a) Dysuria
    (b) Frequency
    (c) Flank pain
    (d) Baseline colony counts of organisms 10^5/ml

11. It is desirable to use a drug whose distribution and excretion are primarily in the urinary tract because:
    (a) Urinary tract infection usually occurs without simultaneous infection elsewhere
    (b) Residual drug that reaches the intestine can alter normal bowel flora and lead to secondary infections
    (c) Drugs with wider distribution tend to be more expensive
    (d) Agents that are urinary-tract specific do not cause nausea or vomiting

Harding et al
12. Resistance to nitrofurantoin during therapy:
    (a) Occurs frequently
    (b) Rarely develops (a statement supported by published accounts over many years of worldwide use)
    (c) May take place by means of plasmid transfer
    (d) Is often a cause of therapeutic failure

13. The authors found nitrofurantoin macrocrystals should remain a first-line therapy of acute, uncomplicated UTIs in women for all but one of the following reasons:
    (a) The cost of therapy is about one third that of norfloxacin
    (b) Nitrofurantoin macrocrystals was as well-tolerated as norfloxacin
    (c) Patients preferred nitrofurantoin macrocrystals
    (d) There was no difference in outcome with the two medications

Brumfitt and Hamilton-Miller
14. Which of the following is *not* a criterion for a low-dose, long-term urinary antibiotic?
    (a) Low cost
    (b) Low incidence of side effects
    (c) Maintenance of continuous antibacterial urinary levels
    (d) No fostering of resistance in bowel flora

15. Which of the following four agents was described by the authors as having a particular advantage in long-term therapy because it is not associated with bacterial resistance?
    (a) Norfloxacin
    (b) Nitrofurantoin macrocrystals
    (c) Trimethoprim/sulfamethoxazole
    (d) Methenamine salts

Van Kerrebroeck
16. "Significant bacteriuria", defined by a quantitative culture obtained by the clean catch technique, is characterized by the following bacterial count:
    (a) 10^6 CFUs/ml
    (b) 10^5 CFUs/ml
    (c) 10^4 CFUs/ml
    (d) 10^8 CFUs/ml

17. The high rate of recurrence in uncomplicated UTIs results from all but one of these factors:
    (a) Failure to comply with the medication regimen
    (b) Poor perineal hygiene
    (c) Excessive frequency of sexual intercourse
    (d) Build-up of bladder bacteria through incomplete voiding

Mulholland
18. After a few days, antimicrobial therapy will sterilize the urine of a patient who has:
    (a) Chronic pyelonephritis
    (b) An uncomplicated reinfection
    (c) Prostatitis
    (d) Stone disease

19. The author prefers nitrofurantoin macrocrystals to cephalexin, trimethoprim, TMP/SMX, and cinoxacin because:
    (a) These other agents have a potentially harmful effect on fecal and vaginal flora
    (b) Nitrofurantoin macrocrystals has a broader antimicrobial spectrum
    (c) Nitrofurantoin macrocrystals causes fewer side effects
    (d) Nitrofurantoin macrocrystals is much less expensive

Nickel

20. Aggressive screening examination of a child with UTI includes all but:
    (a) Intravenous pyelogram
    (b) Renal ultrasonography
    (c) Voiding cystourethrogram
    (d) Cystoscopy

21. Urinary catheterization achieves all but one of the following objectives:
    (a) Relieves temporary urinary obstruction
    (b) Facilitates surgical repair of the urethra and surrounding structures
    (c) Helps prevent infection
    (d) Provides a dry environment for comatose or incontinent patients

Elhilali

22. Recurrence of uncomplicated UTI should lead to the following course of action:
    (a) Change antibiotics
    (b) Try a second course of the original antibiotic
    (c) Consider urethral dilatation
    (d) Prescribe a course of steroids

23. The "urethral syndrome" consists of:
    (a) Recurrent or persistent symptoms, with sterile urine
    (b) Sexually-related UTI episodes
    (c) Structurally-related urinary tract infection
    (d) All episodes of lower urinary tract infection

ANSWER CARD

Please print

Name _____

Address _____
                No. and Street

_____
City   State   Zip

Please circle your answers on this card and return to:

Division of Continuing Education
Bowman Gray School of Medicine
Wake Forest University
300 South Hawthorne Road
Winston-Salem, NC 27103

1.	a	b	c	d	13.	a	b	c	d
2.	a	b	c	d	14.	a	b	c	d
3.	a	b	c	d	15.	a	b	c	d
4.	a	b	c	d	16.	a	b	c	d
5.	a	b	c	d	17.	a	b	c	d
6.	a	b	c	d	18.	a	b	c	d
7.	a	b	c	d	19.	a	b	c	d
8.	a	b	c	d	20.	a	b	c	d
9.	a	b	c	d	21.	a	b	c	d
10.	a	b	c	d	22.	a	b	c	d
11.	a	b	c	d	23.	a	b	c	d
12.	a	b	c	d					